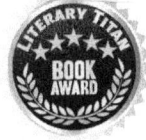

THE
VITALITY
Solution

**Recharge your health with IV Vitamin Therapy,
Mindfulness, Fasting, and more!**

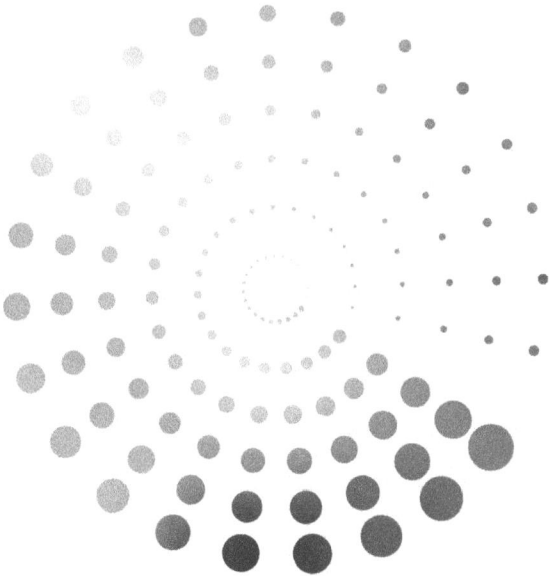

CAREY MENCARINI
Foreword by Aurora Winter, MBA

the vitality solution

RECHARGE YOUR HEALTH WITH IV VITAMIN THERAPY, MINDFULNESS, FASTING, AND MORE!

CAREY MENCARINI

LIV
OPTIMAL

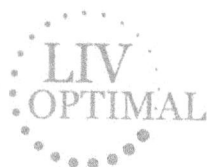

Publication date: May 14, 2024
ISBN: 978-1-966419-00-6 e-book
ISBN: 978-1-966419-01-3 softcover
ISBN: 978-1-966419-02-0 hardcover

praise for the vitality solution

"The Vitality Solution is a compelling read for anyone interested in alternative health, especially those who feel let down by conventional medicine. If you're dealing with chronic illness, unexplained symptoms, or just looking to optimize your health naturally, this book offers both inspiration and actionable steps. Mencarini's firsthand experience and unwavering belief in the body's ability to heal make this book an engaging and motivating guide to wellness."

-LITERARY TITAN 5-STAR REVIEW

"A beacon of hope for chronic illness sufferers. Mencarini's story and strategies offer a path to renewed vitality and well-being."

- JANET BAILEY, PHD

"Carey's personal journey and professional expertise combine to create a compelling roadmap for holistic health and healing."

- HA DANG, ND LAC

"The Vitality Solution is jam-packed with information and ways to regain your health in a more informed and natural way!"

- BRITTNEY STEWART, RN

To my husband, Mike, and my two boys,
Nick and Austin.

You are the air I breathe; you were my willpower
when I had none, my reason for enduring
and persevering when I wanted to give up.

The years of uncertainty, the many 911 calls,
ER visits and hospital stays would have broken
many a family, but your strength and
unwavering steadfastness gave me
the strength to go on.

I thank God every day for blessing my life
with such amazing men!

contents

foreword

BY AURORA WINTER

When Carey Mencarini first shared her health journey with me, I was deeply moved. After facing life-threatening health challenges and being told she had mere months to live, Carey refused to give up. Her determination led her to explore alternative therapies, and today she stands before us radiant, vibrant, and healthier than ever—a testament to the power of perseverance and holistic health practices.

It was with great excitement that I collaborated with Carey using my Spoken Author™ method to bring her mission to life through this book. The result is a culmination of her hard-won knowledge, combining personal experience with professional expertise. Recently, I experienced firsthand the effectiveness of Carey's recommendations when they helped me overcome a virus in just days, while family members with the same illness struggled for weeks.

This isn't just a book to read; it's a road map to a healthier, more vibrant you. The information here has the potential to help you feel younger, healthier, and more energized. It could also be the lifeline someone needs to rekindle hope and reclaim their birthright of health and happiness.

This book is more than a collection of health tips—it's a lifeline, a beacon of hope, and a guide to living your best life.

Warmly,

Aurora Winter, MBA
Founder, www.SamePagePublishing.com
Bestselling author of *Turn Words Into Wealth*
April, 2025

introduction

This book brings awareness to holistic therapies and natural healing methods that many don't know about. It offers hope to those searching for alternative tools to heal themselves or live longer with vitality. I've been fortunate to experience many of these healing therapies and still use most of them today to support my busy lifestyle. While I don't claim to know everything, I want to open doors of possibility and share the experiences of those—both myself and others—who have walked this path.

I'm passionate about creating awareness and empowering others to take charge of their health. My hope is to provide useful tools, resources, and steps you can take today toward optimal health and longevity. In an age of technological advancement and medical challenges, being proactive about your health has never been more important—or looked more promising.

We're living in a unique moment for health empowerment. Rapid advances in medical science have deepened our understanding of cellular health and healing. Information and tools that were once available only to specialists are now accessible to everyone. Meanwhile, rising health care costs make prevention increasingly crucial, and our changing health care landscape can leave people feeling lost in the system. These shifts create both an urgent need and an unprecedented opportunity to take charge of our own health journey.

This book includes remarkable testimonials from IV Lounge clients and fellow patients who prove that these experiences aren't just personal—they're universal. It's written for anyone who wants to achieve vitality and longevity naturally. If you're tired of endless cycles of illness and disease, or multiplying medications that produce little improvement in your wellness or quality of life, this book is for you. If you're dealing with autoimmune disease, chronic illness, high blood pressure, cholesterol issues, mood or cognitive challenges, or simply seeking anti-aging tools that promote vibrant longevity, I hope to spark your interest!

The information in this book does not constitute medical advice, and it is no substitute for doctor's recommendations. But it prompts important conversations about options when there seem to be none, and it offers hope to those suffering needlessly as I once did.

I was blessed to have some medical knowledge before I became ill, which helped me distinguish between helpful and harmful approaches to care. And my passion for natural alternatives led me down this path—one that literally saved my life. I've always been fascinated by the body's remarkable ability to heal itself, and by what happens at the cellular level during illness. I am constantly educating myself on various healing modalities and health topics.

Western medicine excels at acute care: handling broken bones, treating physical anomalies, and performing lifesaving interventions. We have brilliant doctors and institutions in the United States. Yet many seek care elsewhere due to costs or other restrictions. In my experience, our system often overlooks the power of the human body and mind. It frequently dismisses nutrition's role and overlooks how optimizing basic cellular needs —naturally—can be more effective than prescribing pharmaceuticals that the body may treat as foreign.

My passion is helping people help themselves. Self-reliance is our best defense and prevention in this age of super-viruses, medication shortages, and challenged medical systems. If I can help even one person, my journey and my dad's senseless death won't have been in vain.

You have options. No one can write your story unless you allow it! Even if you read nothing else in this book, I hope this message sinks in.

Every day offers a fresh start; failure only comes from not trying again. Make today the day you prioritize your health. If you can't do it for yourself, do it for those you love! Only our own limiting beliefs hold us back. Your body's ability to heal surpasses what anyone has led you to believe.

Health is the ultimate wealth. Invest in yourself daily and watch the dividends of vitality pay off!

—AUTHOR UNKNOWN

my health journey

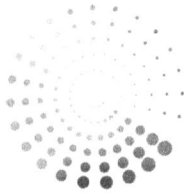

At 45 years old, I was in a wheelchair, on oxygen, and told I was dying. I had two active, growing boys, an amazing husband, a loving family and friends I adored.

Before my health decline, my life could not have been more perfect. I was the owner of a growing photography business, an active leader in the church and a full-time mom running kids around. I was in the prime of my amazing life.

What followed was five years of bizarre symptoms, random diagnoses and hundreds of thousands of dollars spent going to doctors, hospitals and clinics everywhere, in and out of the country. I was finally diagnosed with late-stage neuroborreliosis (Lyme disease) and four co-infections to go with it. It was going to be a long road.

After almost two years of numerous treatments, my body began to shut down and my muscles began to fail. This was when I was diagnosed with nonspecific ALS and handed my death sentence.

How, I wondered, did I get to the point of being incapacitated? Of just *existing*? I thought, "This can't be my life, right?" This so-called death sentence was not acceptable to a driven, type A person like me, and I wasn't about to concede. I knew God had a plan for me. I just had to figure it out.

After allowing myself a small pity party—it is important to grieve before you can move on—I pulled up my bootstraps and went to work, trying to find some resemblance of health in alternative therapies. I knew I had to keep myself alive somehow, so I decided to go back to basics: nutrition.

Due to my inability to swallow or digest food, I turned to IV nutrient therapy and daily hydration, which literally kept me alive. Eventually, we found a doctor who listened and took the time to dig into my three-inch binders—four of them, to be exact—full of tests and records of hospital and doctor visits.

While we were searching for some kind of answer to my predicament, I tried numerous Western treatments, diets and therapies, but nothing seemed to help my muscle deterioration. A piece of the puzzle was missing. Then my doctor noticed that a brain MRI that had been done four years prior showed a Chiari malformation. The malformation was slight, but enough to prevent most of my cerebrospinal fluid from reaching my brain.

On December 12, 2012—an auspicious 12-12-12—I had brain surgery that saved my life. The next day I could walk mostly on my own, and I could breathe again. As my muscles began to get the oxygen and nutrients they needed, I became strong enough to treat my Lyme disease, which was still an issue. Over the course of three years, I dove deeper into alternative medicine and began aggressive treatments. All the while, I conjured the idea of starting a nutrient IV bar to help others. Now that I was finally healing my body, I became very passionate about helping others do the same with alternative practices like IV nutrient therapy.

I am happy to report that, as I write this today, I am healthier than I've been in a long time and full of vitality. To be here with my loving family and friends, to walk and talk and breathe on my own, is an immense blessing. I thank God for every day. And it's a blessing I want to pass on by bringing awareness to alternative approaches to health care and *healing*.

The number of people struggling with chronic illness, disease, cancer or mental health issues is staggering. Never in our history has it been more important to be aware of your choices when it comes to healing. Few people understand the power of natural alternatives. Our bodies are amazingly designed to heal themselves when given the right tools. And as the alternative health movement grows, more people will understand that our power to heal really lies within ourselves and the choices we make every day.

I pray you find what you are looking for and that you allow no one else to write your story! You are here for a reason and loved beyond words. Where your mind is, your body will follow, so be kind to yourself and others. If this girl can make it out of the deepest wilderness, *anyone* can.

Disappointments are inevitable; discouragement is a choice.

—CHARLES STANLEY

a heart-to-heart about this book

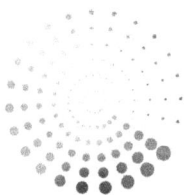

Before we dive into healing and vitality, I want to have an honest conversation with you. The information in this book comes from my thirty-plus years of personal experience—both as a patient and as a professional in various medical roles. Before chronic illness redirected my path, I was finishing pre-med courses for nursing school at night while being a full-time mom, driven by my lifelong passion for helping others.

My fascination with the human body has led me to spend countless hours studying and learning. I've taken many courses, earned certifications, attended webinars, and explored various healing methods. Along the way, I've connected with respected professionals in both alternative and conventional medicine.

Having experienced both the benefits and limitations of conventional medicine, I found myself drawn to alternative healing approaches. Let me be clear—I deeply respect many of the doctors and medical institutions I've worked with and been treated by. Every aspect of medicine serves a purpose. However, few people understand or have been exposed to alternative medicine's gentler approach, which works *with* your body's natural healing abilities rather than against them.

I'm writing this book to share what I've learned. At work and in my personal life, people often ask for my insights, and many have encouraged me to write this book. While I don't enjoy talking about myself—this book isn't meant to be an autobiography—I'll share parts of my journey when they might offer hope to others. My goal is to introduce you to alternative therapies that I've found crucial for anyone facing chronic illness or disease.

This book touches on various aspects of healing and shows how to support your body's needs and identify what might be blocking your path to wellness. I hope it will inspire those who are struggling and desperately seeking any ray of hope—those who feel, as I once did, that they are out of options.

I'll say it again because it's important: this is not medical advice. My purpose is to spark conversations about little-known alternative healing possibilities. Though illness redirected my path away from becoming a doctor, I hope sharing my journey and knowledge will bless those who read this. If this book helps even one person, it will make my life-altering experiences, near-death moments, and sacrifices worthwhile.

immunity
UNLOCKING YOUR HEALING POTENTIAL

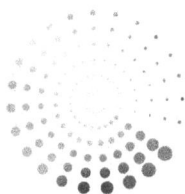

"In any given moment we have two options: to step forward into growth or to step back into safety."

—ABRAHAM MASLOW

Our immune system is a marvel of nature, quietly protecting us day and night. Yet, we often take it for granted until it falters. In this chapter, we'll explore how you can harness your body's innate healing abilities and boost your immunity naturally. We will look at ways that we can influence our DNA, our digestive system (or gut), and also the impact of stress has on our immune system. I will also share the benefits—some obvious and others not so obvious—of boosting our immunity. As someone who's navigated her own health challenges, I'm excited to share insights that could help you transform your well-being.

GENETICS VS. LIFESTYLE: YOU'RE IN CONTROL

Many believe our genes dictate our health destiny, but that's only part of the story. While we can't change our genetic code, we have tremendous power over how those genes express themselves through our lifestyle choices. This is called epigenetics, and it is at the forefront of research today.

Recent research suggests a fascinating discovery: "Nonheritable influences, particularly microbes, seem to play a huge role in driving immune variation," says Dr. Mark Davis, professor of microbiology and director of Stanford's Institute for Immunity, Transplantation and Infection. Davis explains that our immune system adapts to various environmental factors, a process that can overshadow genetic influences. Our DNA does not control our destiny.

Think of it this way: your genes might load the gun, but your lifestyle choices pull the trigger. This means you have more control over your health than you might think! Your grandparents' or even your parents' health history is not your destiny.

If certain health issues run in your family, consider it a heads-up rather than a life sentence. Use this knowledge as motivation to be proactive about your health. By avoiding known triggers and adopting healthy habits, you can often prevent or manage symptoms without relying solely on medication.

THE GUT-BRAIN-IMMUNE CONNECTION: YOUR INTERNAL ECOSYSTEM

The gut-brain axis, as it is commonly called, is connected by millions of nerves, most importantly the vagus nerve. In fact, it is so important that our gut has been dubbed our "second brain." The links between digestion, mood, health and the way we think are strong—and that means what we do with our gut is important.

You've probably heard the saying "Let food be thy medicine" or "All disease begins in the gut." This ancient wisdom from Hippocrates, who was considered the father of modern medicine (and who, by the way, *focused on holistic health care*) is more relevant today than ever. But how does what we eat affect our overall health?

Imagine your gut as a bustling city, home to trillions of microbes. These tiny residents play a crucial role in your health, directly influencing everything from your immune function to your mood. New research indicates that people with a healthy and diverse set of microbes are less likely to suffer from anxiety and depression. In fact, it is believed that 80% of your immune cells reside in the gut lining. Taking care of it is *vital* to your health and your mind.

The Standard American Diet (SAD), unfortunately, is like a wrecking ball in this delicate ecosystem. Packed with inflammatory foods, it can compromise your gut's ability to absorb nutrients, leading to a host of health issues over time.

But here's the good news: gastrointestinal restoration is possible. By making mindful food choices, you can nurture your gut microbiome and, in turn, boost your immunity and overall well-being. A diet that consists mostly of whole foods like vegetables, fruits, legumes, nuts, and seeds can have a profound effect on your microbiome. These foods are packed with fiber, which feeds your beneficial gut bacteria, and antioxidants that combat inflammation. Feeding our gut keeps things like leaky gut syndrome (open junctions in the stomach lining that allow food byproducts into our bloodstream) out of the picture, which in turn helps prevent illness and disease.

Now, I'm not suggesting perfection. The key is to be aware of what you eat, to find a balance that works for you, and to listen to your body. Even small changes can make a big difference. Why not challenge yourself to a one- or two-week plant-based experiment and see how you feel?

IMMUNE SYSTEM STRESSORS: IDENTIFYING THE CULPRITS

Our modern lifestyle, while convenient, throws many challenges at our immune system. Let's look at three major stressors.

1. Chronic Stress

Imagine your body is a car. Stress is like constantly revving the engine without ever letting off the gas. Over time, this takes a toll. Chronic stress can impair digestion, suppress immune function, and slow down healing. It's not just in your head—it affects every cell in your body.

2. *Poor Sleep*

Sleep isn't just downtime; it's when your body goes into repair-and-restore mode. Poor sleep disrupts this rehabilitation process, leading to increased levels of stress hormones like cortisol, which leads to weight gain and speeds up the aging process. This, in turn, can inhibit your immune system's ability to function optimally.

3. *Toxins*

We're exposed to countless toxins daily, from environmental to chemicals in our food and personal care products. These toxins can interfere with our body's nutrient absorption and trigger immune responses; they can even damage our cells and DNA. While we can't eliminate all toxins, we can take steps to reduce our exposure and support our body's natural detoxification processes.

IMMUNITY: YOUR BODY'S SUPERPOWER

A robust immune system is like having your own superhero team. Here's what a well-functioning immune system can do:

1. **DETECT AND FIGHT OFF INFECTIONS**: Your immune system is constantly on patrol, identifying and neutralizing harmful invaders.
2. **RECOGNIZE "SELF"**: It's smart enough to know which cells belong to you. Protect them from friendly fire.
3. **REMEMBER PAST BATTLES**: Like a seasoned warrior, your immune system keeps a record of previous

infections, so it can respond to threats more quickly in the future.

4. **KNOW WHEN TO STAND DOWN**: Once a threat is neutralized, a healthy immune system can calm its response, preventing unnecessary inflammation.

SUCCESS STORIES: REAL PEOPLE, REAL RESULTS

Alec's Story

Imagine being a wine sommelier who suddenly can't taste or smell—it's like a pianist losing their fingers. That was Alec's nightmare in 2021, when COVID stripped him of the senses his career depended on. After months of trying everything, he walked into our IV Lounge, desperate for help.

We treated him with our Immunity IV that first day. But the real moment of hope came the next morning when Alec called us, his voice trembling with excitement. For the first time in months, he could taste—even if it was just the faint sweetness of Gatorade. It was the first sign his world of flavors might return.

Two more Immunity IV treatments later, Alec had fully recovered his senses. What could have ended his career as a sommelier became instead a powerful reminder of the body's ability to heal with the right support. Today, he's back to distinguishing the subtle notes of fine wines, his livelihood and passion restored.

Nancy's Triumph

Nancy came to us in 2022, worn down by a high-stress job and frequent illnesses. When faced with a serious health challenge, she incorporated our Immunity IVs into her treatment plan with her doctor's approval.

The results were astounding. Nancy navigated her treatments with surprising ease in comparison to other patients at the clinic, recovering faster than she or the doctor expected. Her experience underscores the potential of supporting your body's natural healing abilities, even in the face of significant health challenges.

ACTIONS YOU CAN TAKE TODAY:

Remember, supporting your immune system is an investment in your future health. Here are some practical steps you can take right away:

1. **WHO'S DRIVING**: Remember, you are in control, not your genes.
2. **FOR YOUR MIND & IMMUNITY**: Increase fiber-rich foods and decrease the inflammatory ones.
3. **LIFESTYLE OPTIMIZATION**: Get quality sleep, limit daily stress, and reduce toxin exposure.
4. **KNOW YOUR SUPERPOWER**: Be aware of the signals before your body gets depleted.
5. **MAINTAIN NUTRIENT BALANCE**: Supplement high-quality vitamins daily, as needed.

You have the power to transform your health. Every choice you make is an opportunity to support your immune system and enhance your overall well-being. It's not about perfection—it's about progress. Start with small changes, listen to your body, and celebrate every step forward.

Your journey to vibrant health starts now. You've got this!

I've created something special just for you—beautifully designed Action Cards that capture the essential steps to vibrant health! These premium cards, available as a free PDF, are your daily reminder of the vital practices we've explored. Place them where they'll inspire you most—your fridge, mirror, journal, or car. I'd love to see how you're using yours! Claim your exclusive gift now (limited time offer): www.thevitalitysolutionbook.com/gifts.

"What you put at the end of your fork is more powerful medicine than anything you'll find at the bottom of a pill bottle."

—DR. MARK HYMAN

Don't wait for illness
to start valuing wellness!

-author unknown

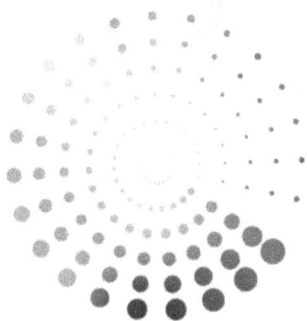

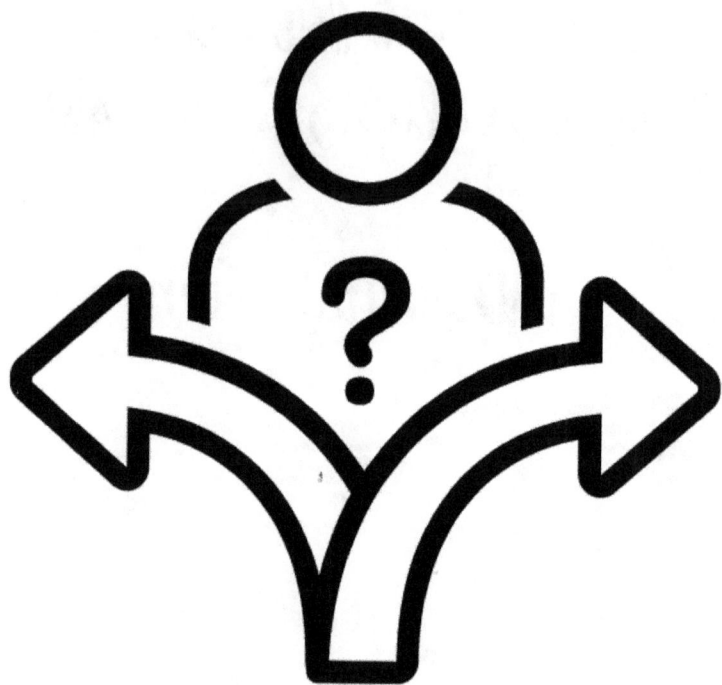

WHO'S DRIVING?

#1

REMEMBER YOU ARE IN CONTROL, NOT YOUR GENES.

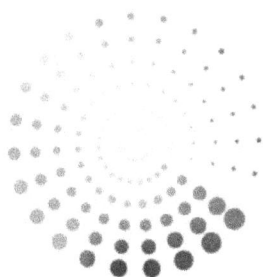

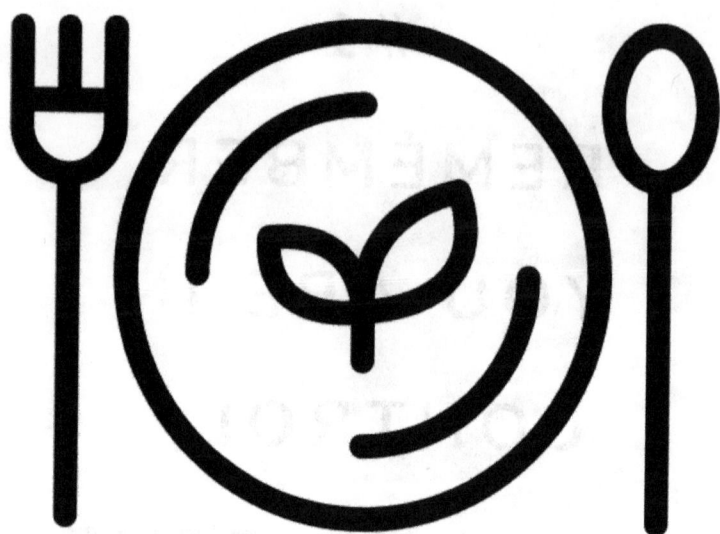

FOR YOUR

MIND & IMMUNITY

#2

INCREASE
FIBER RICH FOODS
& DECREASE THE
INFLAMMATORY
ONES

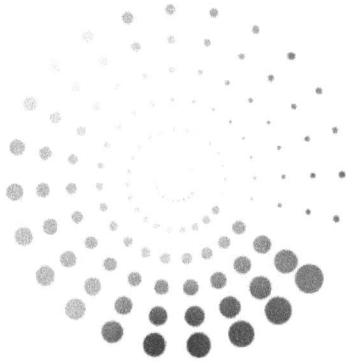

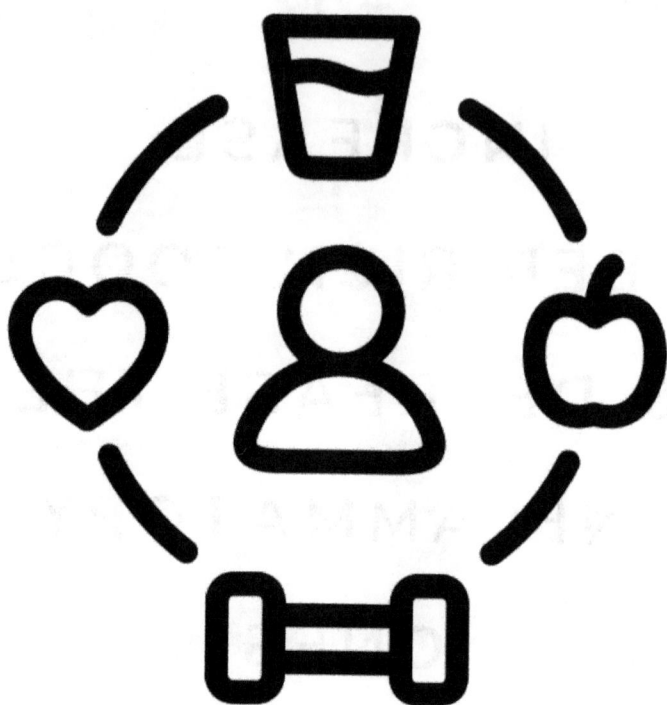

LIFESTYLE
OPTIMIZATION

#3

GET QUALITY SLEEP, LIMIT DAILY STRESS AND REDUCE TOXIN EXPOSURE.

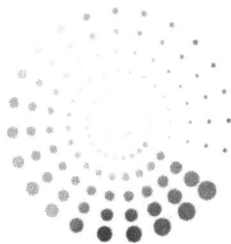

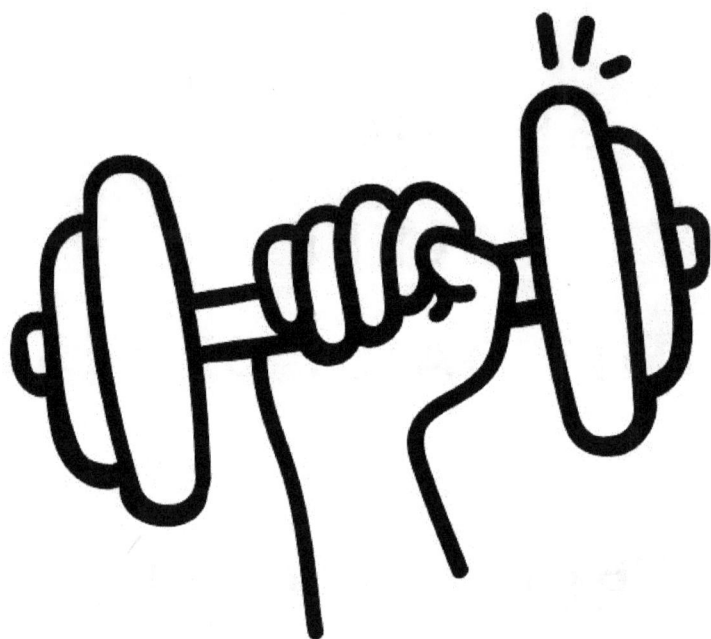

KNOW YOUR

SUPERPOWER

#4

BE AWARE OF THE SIGNALS BEFORE YOUR BODY GETS DEPLETED

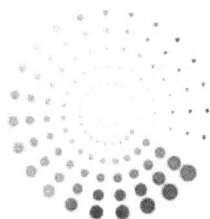

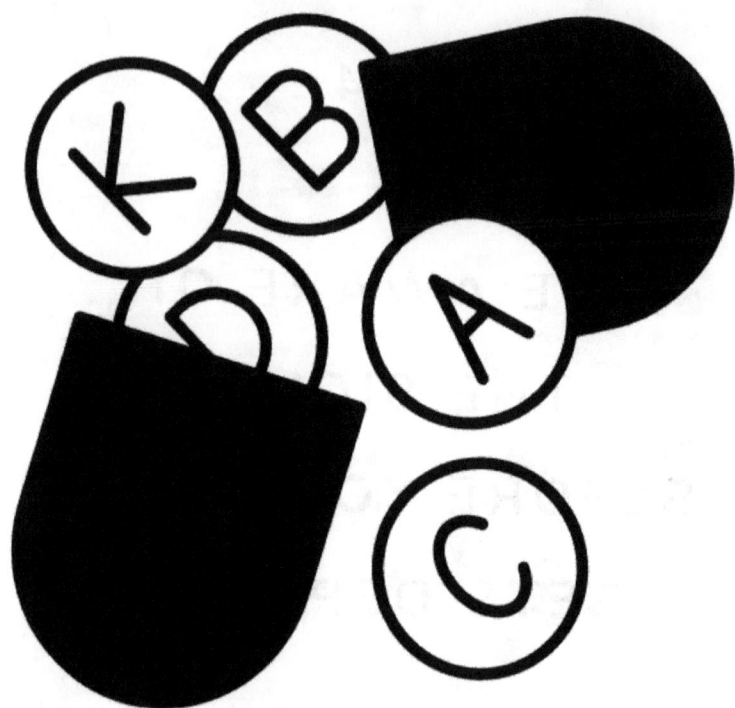

MAINTAIN

NUTRIENT

BALANCE

#5

SUPPLEMENT

HIGH-QUALITY

VITAMINS DAILY,

AS NEEDED.

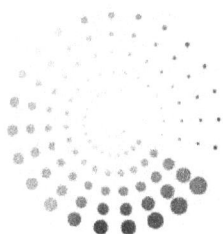

www.the vitalitysolutionbook.com

detoxification

REMOVING THE TOXINS THAT BLOCK HEALTH

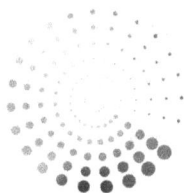

"Our bodies tolerate a fair bit of abuse, however, the less toxins they have to process, the more efficiently they operate."

—KRISSY BALLINGER

When life is good and you're feeling healthy, detoxification might seem unnecessary. But here's the truth: achieving optimal health is impossible without addressing the daily toxins our bodies absorb. In today's world, toxins are more prevalent than ever before. They're in our food, our homes, our personal care products, and even our water. While we can't completely avoid them, we can take steps to minimize their impact on our health.

Fortunately, our bodies are designed to detoxify on a regular basis. This innate process helps maintain homeostasis—the body's state of equilibrium. However, there's a catch. Over the past decade, we've seen a significant increase in the toxins surrounding us. This surge has made it increasingly difficult for our bodies to carry out their natural detoxification processes.

You've likely experienced the effects of ineffective detoxification without even realizing it. Symptoms can include headaches, skin rashes, mood swings, hormonal imbalances, increased susceptibility to colds and flu, fatigue, and brain fog. This list is far from exhaustive. As toxins accumulate over time, they interfere with proper cellular function, overwhelming our systems and leading to unpleasant symptoms.

The consequences of long-term toxin buildup are even more concerning. Toxins that linger in the body can lead to lymphatic congestion and immune system suppression. This state of immunosuppression paves the way for chronic illness, disease, and sometimes cancer. Moreover, this cellular dysfunction accelerates the aging process, affecting both how we feel and how we look.

But don't despair—there's good news. There are simple and effective ways to help our bodies offload these toxins more efficiently. In this chapter, we'll explore several key aspects of detoxification:

1. How we absorb toxins
2. Types of toxins
3. Toxins we need to be aware of
4. Effective methods of detoxification
5. Stages of detox
6. Benefits of detoxing

Understanding these elements is crucial for maintaining good health in our toxin-laden world.

I'll also share my personal detoxification journey and why it became a critical part of my healing process. And you'll read another success story that illustrates the power of detoxification. These real-life examples underscore the importance of addressing toxins at the cellular level to boost your vitality and achieve true health. If we don't remove these toxin roadblocks, we can't effectively heal or attain optimal well-being.

BENEFITS OF REGULAR DETOXIFICATION

You might be surprised by the wide-ranging benefits of regular detoxification. Here are seven key advantages:

1. Decreased inflammation
2. Stronger immune system
3. Improved blood flow
4. Weight loss
5. Stabilized mood
6. Enhanced clarity and brain function
7. Increased stamina

That fourth point—weight loss—often catches people off guard. I know it surprised me when I first learned about it! Here's why it happens: fat cells serve as excellent storage compartments for toxins. When we detox, these cells naturally shrink as they release their toxic contents, contributing to weight loss.

However, detoxification shouldn't be viewed solely as a weight loss strategy. While it can help shed pounds, detoxing alone doesn't address the underlying lifestyle factors that contribute to weight gain. (We'll delve deeper into sustainable lifestyle changes in Chapter 6.)

TYPES OF TOXINS

In this chapter, we'll focus on the growing groups of toxins that we can, to some degree, control to improve our health. These toxins fall into five major categories.

1. Environmental Toxins

Our air is filled with pollutants like carbon monoxide, smoke, chemicals from air fresheners, and various other contaminants. The Environmental Working Group (EWG) conducted a study that found blood samples from newborns contained an average of 287 toxins. And that study was conducted 16 years ago—imagine what the numbers might be today!

2. Water-borne Toxins

You might be shocked to learn that 45% of the nation's tap water, according to a 2023 US geological survey, contains one or more types of chemicals known as "forever" chemicals or PFAs. In fact, studies have shown that even some city water sources contain *upwards* of 267 different chemicals. To check the quality of your local water supply, visit www.EWG.org/tapwater. Hydration is key to maintaining your health, but sometimes the water supply is part of the problem.

3. Food Toxins

Our food supply is laden with toxins. Meats often contain hormones, pesticides, and antibiotics, while fresh produce can be coated with pesticides. The Environmental Working Group reports that a staggering 95% of cancer cases are linked to our environment and diet. Even more alarming, multiple studies have shown that most of us have between 400 and 800 chemical residues stored in our body fat cells. Let that sink in for a moment —up to 800 different chemicals stored in our fat!

For an eye-opening look at this issue, I highly recommend watching the documentary *Food Matters*. While I always approach documentaries and books with a critical eye, it's hard to ignore the film's consistent findings across various reputable sources.

(By the way, I want to ensure you have access to the latest therapies, tools, and research that can support your health journey. I test and validate everything I recommend. For the most up-to-date information, including recommended products, books, movies, trusted companies, current research, upcoming Vitality Solution events, and special promotions, visit: www.thevitalitysolutionbook.com/resources.)

4. Electromagnetic Fields (EMF)

Not all electromagnetic fields are harmful. In fact, our bodies naturally produce weak EMFs. However, it's the frequency (anything measured over 60 hertz) of external EMFs that can be problematic. Here are a few common sources of potentially harmful EMFs:

- Wi-Fi networks
- "Dirty electricity" (spikes and surges above 60 Hz) from power lines or home wiring

- Microwaves
- Cell phones
- Cell towers and power lines

5. Toxins in Personal Care Products

Many of the products we apply to our skin contain harmful chemicals. Here are some common toxins found in personal care items:

1. Sulfates
2. Parabens
3. Phthalates
4. Synthetic colors
5. Artificial fragrances
6. Triclosan
7. Toluene
8. Talc

Navigating the world of toxin-free products can be challenging, but there are great resources available. To get started, visit: https://thevitalitysolutionbook.com/resources.

The key to addressing toxins is awareness, not fear. By educating ourselves, we can make informed choices that protect our health and the health of those we love. In the following sections, we'll explore symptoms of toxin overload and effective detoxification methods to help your body thrive in our modern world.

HOW WE ABSORB TOXINS

Our bodies absorb toxins through three primary pathways:

1. Ingestion
2. Inhalation
3. Absorption through the skin

Understanding these routes of exposure is crucial for developing effective detoxification strategies.

SYMPTOMS OF TOXIN OVERLOAD

Knowing where you fall on the scale of toxin load can help you understand the detoxification that you need. Toxin accumulation can be broken down into three stages:

Stage 1: Acute Phase

This is the body's initial response to toxins, often triggered by new or brief exposures. Symptoms at this stage are the body's natural attempts to eliminate toxins and can include:

- Excessive urination
- Sneezing
- Increased mucus production
- Diarrhea
- Sore throat
- Heartburn
- Nasal congestion
- Occasional vomiting

At this stage, toxins, depending on their type, can often be reduced or eradicated.

Stage 2: Build Up of Over-Accumulation

As toxins build up, you may start experiencing

- Mood swings
- Headaches
- Gastrointestinal issues
- Bloating
- Weight gain
- Brain fog
- Memory issues
- Sleep impairment
- Fatigue
- Depression
- Weakened immunity
- Skin issues, like acne

Stage 3: Toxin Overload

This advanced stage of toxin accumulation has been linked to the development of chronic diseases, autoimmune conditions, and even cancer. At the point of toxin overload, there are more compromised cells than healthy ones in your body.

JESSICA'S STORY: OVERCOMING VIRAL TOXIN OVERLOAD

To illustrate the impact of toxin overload and the power of detoxification, I'd like to share Jessica's story.

Jessica came to IV Lounge as a client, referred by another satisfied customer. She was struggling with lingering symptoms from a COVID-19 infection and, like many long-haul COVID sufferers, couldn't seem to shake them off. Her symptoms were largely due to recirculating toxins left over from the virus that her body wasn't able to eliminate.

While we don't treat specific conditions at IV Lounge, we often see similar symptoms and can make educated guesses about root causes based on our thorough medical intake process and client feedback.

Jessica's chief complaints were persistent fatigue, brain fog, memory issues, and general malaise.

To address these issues, we started Jessica on our Immunity formula. Similar to the "Myers' cocktail" made famous by Dr. John Myers in the 1960s, this IV serves the following purposes:

1. To support the immune system as it deals with lingering toxins
2. To reduce inflammation
3. To boost energy levels
4. To clear brain fog
5. To boost cellular communication.

Some ingredients in the formula also aid the liver in more effectively releasing toxins.

As Jessica detoxified and her symptoms improved, she became so inspired by her recovery that she joined the IV Lounge team as our first Client Concierge. We're blessed and grateful that she, like many others, could heal from such disruptive post-illness symptoms.

ORGANS OF ELIMINATION

Your body has built-in detox mechanisms, as we saw in the Stage 1 (acute phase) symptoms. Each organ system has natural ways to move toxins out, allowing the body to heal. Taking care of these organs, especially the liver, is crucial for maintaining good health. Let's take a closer look at each of these important players in the detoxification process:

Liver

The liver is the primary detoxification organ. It's responsible for:

- Controlling digestion
- Activating enzymes
- Activating immune cells
- Detoxifying the body
- Storing vitamins and glucose
- Regulating fat metabolism

Ensuring optimal liver function is key to efficient detoxification. As we age or deal with conditions that impair our organs' natural functions, they may work less efficiently, making supplementation necessary. Glutathione, for example, a powerful master antioxidant, helps the liver more effectively process cellular debris and fat cells where toxins often hide.

Gallbladder

Located under the liver, the gallbladder stores and releases bile. This greenish-yellow fluid helps break down fats from the food we eat, then moves these waste products into the colon for elimination. Bile is primarily composed of cholesterol, bilirubin, and bile salts.

Kidneys

These two bean-shaped organs, part of the urinary system, sit in the back of your abdomen. Their main functions are:

- Filtering blood
- Removing cellular waste
- Balancing the body's fluids (electrolytes)

Colon

Also known as the large intestine, the colon is part of the gastrointestinal tract. It transports toxins through fecal matter for elimination. Toxins can accumulate in the bowels, leading to various health issues. In some cases, interventions like enemas or colonics may be necessary to assist the elimination process.

Skin

Our skin is often called the body's largest organ, and it's also an excellent indicator of our overall health. It's our best "tattletale" when something's amiss internally. Symptoms like rashes, acne, eczema, and psoriasis are all signs of some kind of cellular dysfunction.

Lungs

Our lungs provide the oxygen that every cell in our body needs to function. They exchange gases as we breathe in and out, helping the body rid itself of carbon dioxide, a waste product of cellular metabolism.

Lymphatic System

While not strictly an organ of elimination, the lymphatic system plays a crucial role in detoxification. It acts as the immune system's superhighway, cleansing the blood of foreign invaders by initiating the body's immune response and creating white blood cells.

Unlike the circulatory system, which has the heart to pump blood, the lymphatic system lacks a central pump. It relies primarily on gravity and muscle movement to circulate lymph fluid. This is why it's imperative to keep this system moving through deep breathing and other modalities, like the Power Plate, to avoid toxin buildup and overload.

DETOX SYMPTOMS

A word to the wise: if you want to avoid an unpleasant detoxification experience, start low and go slow with whatever method you choose. You don't have to feel bad to get good results, but sometimes when you have a significant buildup of toxins to eliminate, you may experience some discomfort. Stay calm and carry on—it will get better!

RAPID DETOX SYMPTOMS

During a rapid detox, you might experience

- Flu-like symptoms
- Low-grade fever
- Nausea
- Skin rash
- Headache

These symptoms are sometimes referred to as Herxheimer or "Herxing" reactions. They're usually the result of a large cellular "die-off" of microorganisms during toxin release.

Supplements known as binders can help manage these symptoms, but it's crucial to have a fully functioning elimination system in order to use them. Without proper elimination, you risk constipation and toxin reentry or reabsorption, which can make matters worse.

Detoxification is a journey, not a race. By understanding how our bodies absorb and process toxins, recognizing the signs of toxin overload, and supporting our natural detoxification organs, we can take significant steps toward improved health and vitality. In the next section, we'll explore various detoxification methods to help you create a personalized strategy for optimal wellness.

DETOX METHODS

There are several ways to support your body's natural detoxification processes. Let's explore some effective methods.

Physical Detoxification

1. **INFRARED SAUNA:** Sweat it out! Studies have shown that persistent toxins readily release through sweat. Infrared saunas can be effective for deep detoxification.

2. **EPSOM SALT BATHS:** This gentle method not only relaxes you after a busy day but also helps unload cellular debris. The magnesium in Epsom salts supports various detox pathways in the body. Certain essential oils can also have added benefits to detoxification. For more information on essential oils, visit: www.thevitalitysolutionbook.com/resources.

3. **IONIC FOOT SPA:** This relaxing foot bath pulls toxins through the 4,000 pores in your feet into ionically charged water. It's a painless and effective way of detoxing. At IV Lounge, we usually combine this with a short session on the Power Plate for enhanced lymphatic movement. At IV Lounge, these foot baths are often followed by a vitamin IV for enhanced benefits of overall wellness. We take out the *bad* and put in the *good*!

4. **GROUNDING:** Also known as "earthing," this involves the skin's direct contact with the earth's surface. Walking barefoot on grass, sand or soil allows our bodies to absorb negatively charged electrons, neutralizing harmful free radicals. These free radicals can cause inflammation, cell damage, and stress, among other issues. However, unless you walk around barefoot, gardening for a living, touching the earth isn't always possible. Grounding pads are an effective alternative. Available as sheets for your bed or as stand-alone pads, they connect to an outlet via a grounding wire. I use both methods to maximize benefits.

5. **PEMF MAT**: Pulsed Electromagnetic Frequency (PEMF) therapy uses good electromagnetic frequencies to restore balance and regulate energy circulation within the body. This technology improves circulatory efficiency, supports heart health, and can even lower blood pressure. I've been using a PEMF mat for over 10 years, both morning and night, for pain management and overall wellness.

6. **CASTOR OIL PACKS:** This gentle detoxification process involves soaking a cloth in castor oil and placing it on the abdomen, over the liver, or over the thyroid area, as directed by a practitioner. Plastic wrap is usually placed over the pack, and a heating pad is then placed over the pack to enhance absorption. These packs can also be used for pain or menstrual relief, digestive health, and skin health.

Lymphatic Stimulation

Moving your lymph system is crucial for effective detoxification. This closed system needs stimulation to open its valves and allow fluid to flow, preventing toxin buildup. Swollen glands often indicate stagnant lymph flow. Here are some ways to keep your lymphatic system moving:

1. **POWER PLATE VIBRATION**: This whole-body vibration platform helps mobilize lymphatic fluid. At IV Lounge, we often use this before an ionic foot spa to help assist the body in the effective movement of toxins.
2. **DRY BRUSHING**: Using a soft-bristled brush, gently brush your skin toward your heart to stimulate lymph flow. Be careful not to brush too aggressively, as this can have the opposite effect.

3. **REBOUNDING:** Jumping on a small trampoline manually pumps lymphatic fluid, promoting detoxification.

4. **MASSAGE:** Toxins can get trapped in connective tissue called fascia. Myofascial release and massage help break down these webs of tissue, eliminating toxin buildup. Massage increases blood flow and helps organs function more efficiently. Yoga can also help open up these channels through gentle stretching.

5. **RAISED BED:** Elevating the head of your bed slightly— by about five degrees—supports lymphatic drainage. This can be combined with lymphatic self-massage techniques for enhanced benefits.

Supplements that can assist with detoxification

1. **GLUTATHIONE:** Known as the body's master antioxidant, glutathione helps unburden the liver and converts fat-soluble toxins into water-soluble forms that can be eliminated through bodily fluids. An IV is a particularly effective way to deliver usable glutathione, as many oral supplements come in forms that the body can't easily utilize.

2. **BINDERS:** Various binding agents can effectively attach to toxins, allowing them to be eliminated through fecal matter. While using binders, it is important to maintain adequate fiber intake and hydration to prevent constipation. Always consult your physician before using binders, as specific toxins may require specific binding agents. Examples of binding supplements are; charcoal, chlorella, bentonite clay, zeolite, psyllium husk, NAC (N-Acetylcysteine) and cilantro.

Health science evolves rapidly, bringing new opportunities for optimal wellness. As your guide on this journey, I continuously research and validate the most effective therapies, tools, and treatments. For my latest findings, research updates, and vetted recommendations, visit www.thevitalitysolutionbook.com/resources. You'll find everything from breakthrough studies to tried-and-true wellness solutions, all tested and proven.

MY PERSONAL STORY: EXTREME DETOX

After being diagnosed with Lyme disease, I underwent 18 consecutive months of treatments targeting five different infections. These drug cocktails were designed to eradicate Borrelia burgdorferi (the primary Lyme pathogen) and four common co-infections.

These IV treatments were expensive, not covered by insurance, and unsupported by the mainstream medical community. My husband or I administered them at home through a chest port, as there was nonconventional support locally available for chronic Lyme patients.

These treatments, while effective at killing harmful pathogens, also affected what healthy cells I had left. The side effects mirrored those of chemotherapy: nausea, vomiting, hair damage and loss, skin rashes, fevers, weight loss, organ damage and tooth enamel destruction, among others. These symptoms resulted from the cellular debris (released endotoxins) that were recirculating in my body post-treatment. As this debris accumulated, it became increasingly toxic, severely impacting my quality of life. Often, just as I began to feel normal, another round of treatment would start, leaving my immune system little time to recover.

Before starting treatment, my doctor's office warned me about potential Herxheimer reactions. "Herxing" occurs when bacterial die-off releases endotoxins into the bloodstream, triggering an immune response that can worsen existing symptoms and create new ones.

I followed all the recommended protocols. I took toxin-binding supplements, adhered to a specific diet, and limited social contact to avoid germ exposure. Despite these efforts, my body struggled to release toxins. I soon learned I had a genetic predisposition that made detoxification extremely challenging. We reduced treatment intensity, hoping it would help, but it was futile.

This experience led me to dive deep into information about detoxification and the tools that could support this process. I knew I was fighting an uphill battle, but I needed to help my body eliminate the cellular debris or I wouldn't be able to continue treatment.

I implemented a comprehensive detox regimen:

- Daily infrared sauna sessions
- Daily Epsom salt baths, or footbaths when moving was painful
- Regular use of a PEMF (pulsed electromagnetic frequency) mat
- Frequent outdoor grounding sessions to neutralize EMFs and negative energy
- Lymphatic stimulation to keep toxins moving and pathways open
- Continued daily prayer and meditation, which have always anchored me during difficult times

I complemented these external methods with internal approaches:

- Daily homemade green juice for liver cleansing
- Supplements to support kidney, spleen, and liver function
- Plenty of water daily to flush toxins and maintain hydration

Hydration is key. The Institute of Medicine's daily recommendation is 125 ounces for men and 91 ounces for women (this includes all fluid intake, not just water). Holistic guidelines recommend two liters a day depending on your activity levels. Adding a pinch of pink Himalayan salt will also help you maintain adequate electrolytes, which help keep water in the cells. Staying hydrated also eases elimination, helps cells function properly, and improves our overall brain function.

Through this journey, I learned that even with genetic challenges, there are always options to support your body's natural detoxification processes. Nothing is impossible; you just need to keep an open mind and be willing to try unconventional approaches that can potentially save your life.

SIGNS YOUR DETOX IS WORKING

As you implement these detoxification strategies, look for the following signs of progress:

- Decreased fatigue and improved sleep
- Fewer digestive issues
- Increased stamina

- Reduced pain or stiffness
- More stable mood
- Enhanced mental clarity and memory
- Stronger immune system
- Overall sense of wellness

ACTIONS YOU CAN TAKE TODAY

1. **KNOW YOUR ENVIRONMENT**: Be mindful of what you ingest, inhale, and absorb.
2. **PAY ATYTENTION TO THE SIGNS**: Listen to your body, pay attention to symptoms of toxin overload.
3. **ENVIRONMENTALLY DETOX**: Filter air/water, eat clean foods and lessen bad EMF's.
4. **INTERNAL DETOX**: Incorporate physical methods of detoxification through various methods and/or supplementation.

Remember, in today's world detoxification is an ongoing process, not a onetime event. By consistently supporting your body's natural detox mechanisms, you're investing in your long-term health and vitality. Start with small, manageable changes and gradually build a detox routine that works for your lifestyle. Your body will thank you for it!

"The body has its own intelligence. Detoxification is a way to support that natural process and promote healing from within."

—DEEPAK CHOPRA

"Our bodies tolerate a fair bit of abuse, however, the less toxins they have to process, the more efficiently they operate."

Krissy Ballinger

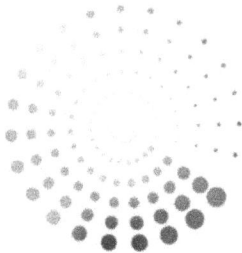

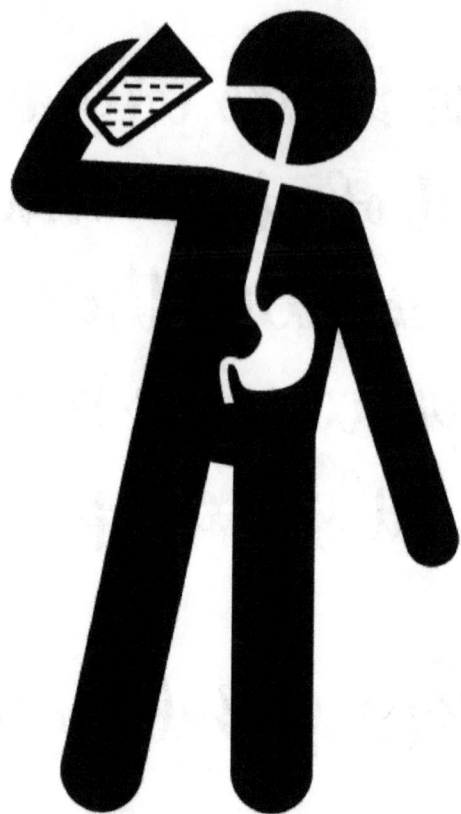

KNOW YOUR
ENVIRONMENT

#1

BE AWARE OF
WHAT YOU INGEST,
INHALE AND
ABSORB,
KNOWLEDGE IS
POWER.

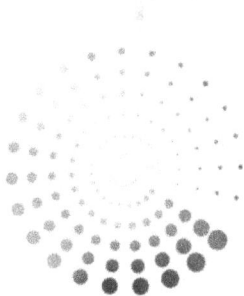

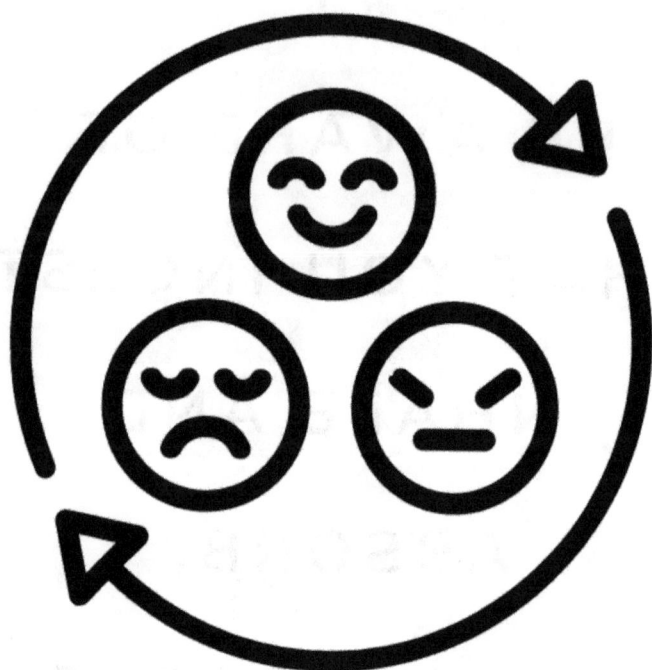

PAY ATTENTION
TO THE SIGNS

#2

LISTEN TO YOUR BODY, PAY ATTENTION TO SYMPTOMS OF TOXIN OVERLOAD.

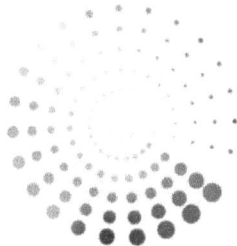

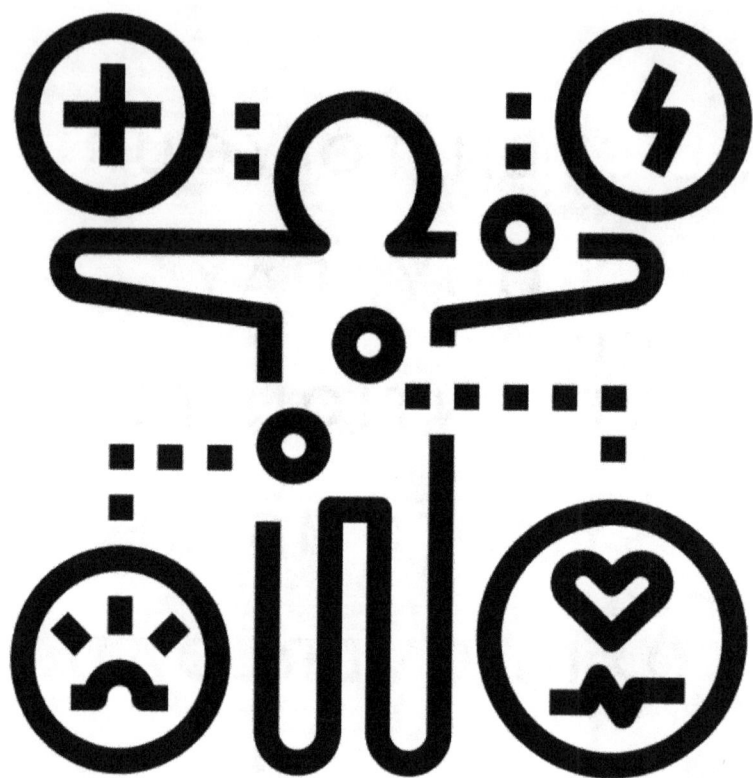

ENVIRONMENTAL
DETOX

#3

FILTER YOUR AIR/WATER, EAT CLEAN FOODS & LESSEN EMF EXPOSURE.

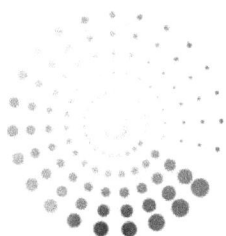

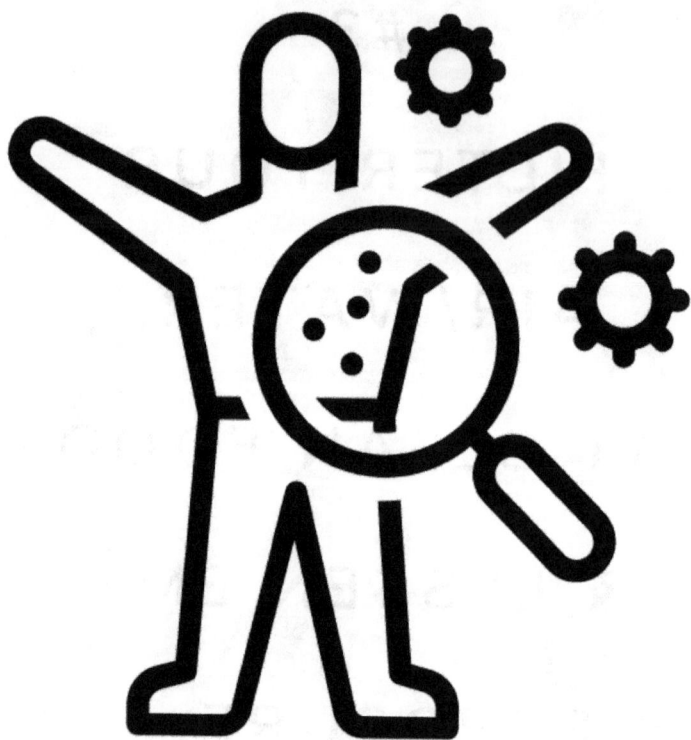

INTERNAL
DETOX

#4

INCORPORATE PHYSICAL METHODS OF DOING DAILY DETOX THROUGH THERAPIES OR SUPPLEMENTS

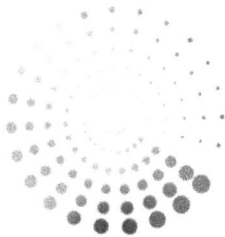

restore

TARGETED CELLULAR NUTRITION

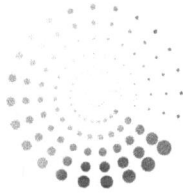

"Time and health are two precious assets that we don't recognize and appreciate until they have been depleted."

—DENIS WAITLEY

Restoring nutrients lost to stress, poor lifestyle choices, illness or disease can be a daunting task. In today's world, we're bombarded with countless vitamin and supplement options, each promising miraculous results. Yet many of these products fall short, leaving us confused and still depleted. When your health is on the line, you need to be certain you're providing your body with the right nutrients at the cellular level.

Welcome to the transformative world of targeted cellular nutrition through intravenous vitamin therapy!! While infusion therapy has been around since the 1800s, it gained significant recognition in the 1960s thanks to Dr. John Myers. His pioneering work with nutrient infusions for patients led to creating the now-famous Myers' cocktail.

It's unfortunate that conventional medicine hasn't yet embraced this powerful therapy. Our society often seems more focused on profiting from illness than preventing it. Just look at the barrage of fast food and pharmaceutical ads during your favorite TV show or sporting event, and the number of hospitals and clinics promoting their services. This trend should make us pause and question where the true priorities in health care lie. Our constant bombardment by these messages is alarming, and it fuels my passion to share health and wellness alternatives. My goal is to empower you with information so you can make informed decisions about your health journey.

Despite these challenging influences, intravenous vitamin therapy is gaining (some well-deserved) popularity. It is becoming accessible to everyone, not just elite athletes and the wealthy. Vitamin infusions have always been, and remain, the most effective method for delivering 100% pharmaceutical-grade vitamins directly to your cells. This approach allows for immediate and efficient replenishment of vital nutrients, building a healthier cellular environment that can help prevent disease and illness.

Even the highest-quality oral vitamins can't compare to IV therapy. Oral supplements require a healthy gut—something many people lack—for proper breakdown and absorption. At best, oral vitamins are absorbed at a fraction of the degree to which infusions are. If you're experiencing ongoing symptoms that impact your daily life—things like brain fog, mood swings, chronic fatigue, insomnia, pain, inflammation, lack of stamina, or dry and wrinkled skin—and you're already taking oral vitamins, the root cause could still be vitamin deficiency and even dehydration.

I can relate to the challenges of maintaining optimal health in our hectic world. My life can be chaotic and demanding, depleting my nutrient reserves without me even realizing it. Some days, no amount of meditation seems to calm my mind, and no food truly fuels my body. As I age, those vital reserves get depleted faster and faster. That's why, as someone with a compromised gut, I rely on regular IV and injection vitamin supplementation to maintain balance and ensure I can accomplish everything on my to-do list. For those dealing with chronic health issues, this kind of cellular support becomes critical just to function.

In previous chapters, we explored how to boost our immune systems and remove the toxin roadblocks that prevent us from achieving optimal cellular health. Now, let's take a closer look at a targeted approach to restoring cells that aren't functioning as effectively as they could be. We'll dive deep into the world of vitamins, examining their benefits to our overall health and the consequences of vitamin deficiencies.

DISEASE OR DEFICIENCY?

We often live life with abandon, taking for granted our body's need for basic nutrition and hydration. Then, out of nowhere, our reserves are drained. Symptoms we've never experienced before become part of our daily routine. The next thing we know, we're sitting in a doctor's office, wondering what went wrong. Or worse, we're told these new symptoms might be early warnings of a chronic illness or disease.

It may seem drastic to go from feeling healthy to facing a dire diagnosis. But this scenario illustrates how adept we've become at tuning out our body's signals. We expect our bodies to function flawlessly on minimal fuel—or, worse, on low-quality fuel. We rarely take the time to investigate potential issues until we're unable to power through our day. By then, we're left wondering why we have all these symptoms and struggle to complete basic tasks.

Human nature drives us to seek the quickest fix for our discomfort. We want to continue on our merry way without looking back to uncover the root cause of our problems. Western medicine often caters to this desire, leading us from one pill to another without addressing the core reasons behind our symptoms.

I don't fault some doctors for this Band-Aid approach to patient care. After all, it's what many patients demand—a quick fix. I've certainly had moments where I wished for a magic pill to make everything better. Who has time to deal with underlying causes when you could eliminate the symptom with medication? The sad reality, however, is that bypassing the root cause behind our symptoms only leads us from one health crisis to another.

But what if these symptoms are signs of vitamin deficiencies? Why not try targeted nutrition first and save pharmaceuticals as a last resort? Unlike medications, vitamins don't come with a laundry list of side effects. Their sole purpose is to support cellular health. The worst outcome of taking vitamins is that you end up feeling hydrated and energized—two things most of us would love to feel more often!

For those who are severely depleted, of course, it may take time to replenish lost reserves. Among those who choose the efficient route of vitamin infusions, some notice a difference after the first IV, while others require several IVs before they notice decreased symptoms or enhanced vitality. The role of adequate cellular nutrition in homeostasis cannot be overstated.

When we allow ourselves to become vitamin deficient, we set ourselves up for a host of health complications, including illness and disease. Once you're running on empty, not only will your valuable time be consumed by doctor appointments and medication management, but your finances will take a hit as well. Suddenly, preventative nutrition looks far more appealing, doesn't it?

Here are some vitamin deficiencies that are often mistaken for more serious illnesses or diseases:

- Peripheral neuropathy: caused more often by a deficiency and in rare cases by an excess of vitamin B6
- anemia: caused by a deficiency of iron
- Osteoporosis: caused by a deficiency of calcium
- Rickets: caused by a deficiency of vitamin D, calcium and potassium
- Pellagra: caused by a deficiency of vitamin B_3 (niacin)
- Scurvy: caused by a deficiency of vitamin C
- Xerophthalmia (night blindness): caused by a deficiency of vitamin A
- Goiter: caused by an iodine deficiency
- Hemorrhage: caused by a deficiency of vitamin K
- Hyperkeratosis: caused by a deficiency of vitamin A
- *Important note: These vitamin deficiencies are not responsible for any illness or disease, but they can be a significant contributing factor. Always consult with your doctor before starting any supplementation regimen.*

GINA'S STORY: OVERCOMING PERIPHERAL NEUROPATHY

A hardworking self-employed entrepreneur—I'll call her Gina—came to us suffering from severe peripheral neuropathy.

The severity of her symptoms fluctuated unpredictably. The pharmaceuticals prescribed by her doctor offered little relief, and, worse, the constant pain was disrupting her sleep, leaving her immune system compromised. Feeling depleted and run down, she found herself vulnerable to every flu bug circulating through her office.

Faced with limited options, Gina's doctor recommended TENS (transcutaneous nerve stimulation) therapy or even surgery if her condition didn't improve. Neither of those felt like viable solutions to her. Determined to find an alternative, Ginadiscovered IV Lounge. In a last-ditch effort to alleviate her constant pain, she scheduled an appointment for an Immunity IV.

The results were remarkable. After just one IV session, Gina experienced less pain and a noticeable boost in energy. Elated by this improvement, she returned the following week for another Immunity IV, this time adding a vitamin D injection to further bolster her immune system. The combined approach proved even more effective.

Gina shared her story on social media, celebrating her newfound relief from years of chronic pain. She became a regular member of our IV Club, committed to maintaining her stronger, more resilient immune system. Today, Gina's schedule is busier than ever, but her cells are now nourished and capable of supporting her active lifestyle.

Note: As of July 2024, vitamin D injections are no longer legally available in California.

THE ORIGIN OF *LIMEYS*: A LESSON IN NUTRITIONAL HISTORY

Have you ever wondered about the origin of the term *limey* to describe a British sailor? This nickname stems from a crucial nutritional discovery. Between the sixteenth and eighteenth centuries, about two million sailors died from scurvy, a disease that could decimate entire ship crews. In the nineteenth century, the British Navy made a groundbreaking decision: they began storing limes and lemons aboard all their ships.

Why citrus? These fruits are rich in vitamin C, which prevents scurvy. American sailors, who were less informed about these preventative measures, dubbed their British counterparts "Limeys" because of their consumption of limes. Little did they know this simple dietary addition was saving lives!

THE RISE OF IV VITAMIN THERAPY

Today, an impressive 86% of adults in the United States take oral vitamin supplements. But many of those who were taking oral supplements are turning to vitamin infusion therapy to enhance their vitality. Why? Because IV therapy offers superior quality, reliability, and effectiveness compared to traditional supplements. This powerful nutritional tool helps people fuel their busy lifestyles, making their bodies more resistant to stress and illness. They're able to function at a higher level every day, and they spend less time missing work or life events due to illness.

IV vitamin therapy offers many benefits beyond immune system support. One of its key advantages lies in its delivery method. By bypassing the digestive system, IV therapy allows for about 99.9% cellular absorption of nutrients. These vital compounds are delivered directly to the bloodstream, reaching the cells that need them most for immediate use. Oral vitamins, in comparison, can take minutes to hours to break down in the gut, and the body typically absorbs or uses less than 20% of their vitamin content.

For those with serious digestive conditions, Vitamin IV therapy can be a game changer. It ensures they receive the nutrition their bodies desperately need, even when traditional absorption methods fail.

JANET'S STORY: OVERCOMING GI MALABSORPTION

Janet Bailey has been a loyal IV Lounge client since we opened our doors. Years ago, she underwent gastric bypass surgery, which significantly reduced the size of her stomach and intestines. While this helped with weight loss, it left her body struggling to absorb nutrients from both food and oral vitamins.

For years, Janet battled the consequences of nutrient deficiency: crushing fatigue, persistent brain fog, disrupted sleep, mood swings, digestive issues, and a weakened immune system. She seemed to catch every virus going around, which interfered with her work and overall enjoyment of life. Despite losing weight, Janet was far from healthy. These symptoms of vitamin insufficiency are common among those who've undergone bariatric surgery.

In 2021, Janet began receiving our Immunity formula. The transformation was remarkable. She regained her energy and mental clarity. Her sleep improved, and she became more resilient to viruses. Overall, Janet was functioning better than she had in years.

Over the past two years, Janet has graduated to our NAD IV formula. This advanced treatment builds on the benefits of the Immunity formula while adding powerful anti-aging benefits and optimizing cellular energy and repair processes. To maintain her progress between monthly IV sessions, Janet uses our NAD NITRO injections. This combination keeps her energy levels high, her immune system strong, and her cellular health at its peak.

Today, Janet is thriving. She has more stamina than ever. Her cells are repairing themselves at an accelerated rate. Even environmental toxins and everyday stressors that used to slow her down are now easier for her to manage. Janet is living with a level of vitality and youth she once only dreamed of experiencing again.

ESSENTIAL NUTRIENTS AND THEIR DEFICIENCIES

Let's explore some essential vitamins and the impact their deficiencies can have on our health.

Vitamin B$_{12}$ (Cobalamin)

This water-soluble vitamin is crucial for blood formation, brain function and nerve health. Methylcobalamin is the most bioavailable form, which means it's easier for your body to use. Every cell in your body relies on B$_{12}$ to function properly, but here's the catch—your body can't produce it on its own. You must get B_{12} through diet or supplements.

Vitamin B_{12} is primarily found in animal-based foods. While some seaweed and plant sources offer small amounts, those following vegan or plant-based diets (like me) are at higher risk of deficiency. Studies indicate that up to 80 to 90% of vegetarians and vegans are deficient in vitamin B.

Symptoms of B_{12} deficiency include weakness, dizziness, pale skin, shortness of breath, nerve problems, poor memory or concentration, diarrhea, anemia, and other blood disorders.

It's not just plant-based eaters at risk, though. Over 20% of older adults may be B_{12} deficient due to decreased absorption as we age. As mentioned previously, not all B_{12} is the same; some forms are less bioavailable than others. At IV Lounge, we only provide our clients with the most absorbable form, methylcobalamin.

Other risk factors for B_{12} deficiency include gastritis, ingestion of medications that interfere with B_{12} absorption, and some neurological disorders.

NAD (Nicotinamide Adenine Dinucleotide)

This coenzyme is found in every cell of our bodies. It plays a crucial role in energy production, DNA repair and maintenance, and inflammation management.

As we age, our natural NAD production declines. Scientists believe this decrease is linked to the aging process and may contribute to neurodegenerative conditions.

But NAD isn't just about fighting aging. It can also aid in muscle recovery and help regulate metabolic disorders.

Here are a few signs of NAD deficiency:

- Neurodegeneration
- Brain fog and memory issues
- Confusion
- Muscle weakness and poor recovery
- Sleep disturbances
- Dull, lackluster skin
- Increased oxidative stress (cellular toxins)
- Premature fine lines and wrinkles

Glutathione: The Master Antioxidant

Known as the "Master Antioxidant," glutathione is a powerful amino acid that shields cells from oxidative damage. It plays a crucial role in DNA repair and boosts immune function. This versatile compound intercepts and neutralizes toxins in the gut while aiding liver detoxification, ensuring optimal organ function.

Here are a few signs of glutathione deficiency:

- Persistent fatigue or lack of energy
- Sleep disturbances
- Brain fog
- Weakened immunity and frequent illnesses
- Joint and muscle pain

Vitamin C: A Multifaceted Nutrient

This water-soluble vitamin is a powerhouse of health benefits. It acts as a potent antioxidant, reduces inflammation, enhances immune function, promotes wound healing, and helps prevent iron deficiency.

Early symptoms of vitamin C deficiency:

- Weakness and fatigue
- Sore arms and legs
- Easy bruising and rashes
- Bleeding gums and increased tooth mobility
- Fragile skin
- Unusual hair growth patterns
- Slow-healing wounds
- Joint pain and inflammation

Late-stage symptoms of vitamin C deficiency:

- Decreased red blood cell count
- Gum disease
- Hair loss, luster, or growth
- Skin bleeding
- Bone and blood vessel complications

Magnesium: The Cellular Powerhouse

Magnesium is a key mineral involved in hundreds of enzymatic reactions throughout the body. It's essential for strengthening bone and teeth structure and plays a vital role in many cellular functions.

Alarmingly, about 70% of Americans in the general population consume less than the required amount of magnesium. Low magnesium levels are associated with several health concerns, including type 2 diabetes, metabolic syndrome, heart disease and osteoporosis.

Symptoms of magnesium deficiency:

- Irregular heart rhythms
- Muscle cramps
- Restless leg syndrome
- Fatigue
- Migraines

Long-term, subtle symptoms may include insulin resistance and high blood pressure.

Vitamin D: The Sunshine Vitamin

Vitamin D is a fat-soluble vitamin that functions like a steroid hormone. It travels through your bloodstream, influencing gene expression in cells throughout your body. Nearly every cell has a receptor for vitamin D. This crucial nutrient also aids calcium and phosphorus absorption, supporting strong bones.

Our bodies produce vitamin D when our skin is exposed to sunlight. However, those living far from the equator may be at risk of deficiency without adequate dietary intake or supplementation.

In the United States, vitamin D deficiency is surprisingly common. About 42% of the general population is deficient, and this proportion rises to 74% among older adults and a staggering 82% among people with darker skin tones. No wonder illness and disease is so prevalent today!

Here are a few symptoms of vitamin D deficiency:

- Muscle weakness
- Bone loss
- Weakened immunity
- Increased risk of cancer and fractures
- In children, growth delays and soft bones (rickets)

RESTORING NUTRIENT BALANCE

Our bodies possess an incredible ability to heal themselves when given the right conditions, nutrients and environment. Unfortunately, the Standard American Diet (SAD) and modern lifestyle choices have inadvertently switched off many of our natural healing mechanisms, leaving us vulnerable to illness and disease.

The effectiveness of vitamin supplementation has been debated for centuries. While government guidelines for vitamin intake and a balanced diet are a good starting point, it's important to remember that they are general recommendations. Many people take these guidelines as absolute truth, which can create a false sense of security about their nutritional status. In reality, our vitamin and mineral needs can fluctuate daily based on our lifestyle, health status and dietary choices.

UNDERSTANDING DAILY NUTRIENT RECOMMENDATIONS

The government's Recommended Daily Allowance (RDA) and Recommended Daily Intake (RDI) guidelines represent the minimum required to prevent diseases like scurvy. However, these amounts are quite low by today's nutritional science standards.

Instead of focusing on merely preventing deficiency diseases, we should aim to absorb the optimal amount of vitamins our bodies need to thrive. Drawing upon thousands of studies, researchers have developed Nutrient Reference Values (NRVs) to indicate the daily amount of nutrients required for optimal health. These values can vary based on your location, so it's worth researching the NRVs specific to your region.

It's crucial to understand that if you're taking oral supplements, you're likely only absorbing a fraction of the nutrients compared to the superior IV delivery method. It is important to point out that there are some delivery methods which are more effective than others, such as the liposomal method. The intravenous delivery allows for complete absorption directly into the bloodstream, where nutrients can be immediately utilized by your cells. For those dealing with severe depletion, there's simply no comparison between oral and IV supplementation.

Following the basic governmental guidelines for daily supplementation offers a one-size-fits-all approach. However, our individual needs can vary dramatically from day to day and person to person. No two individuals have identical nutritional requirements.

While you can start with standard guidelines like RDA/RDI and NRV, it's essential to consider the many factors that can influence your body's ability to absorb and utilize nutrients.

FACTORS INFLUENCING VITAMIN ABSORPTION

Think you could be deficient? Here are some factors that could rob you of essential nutrients necessary for good health. How many of these factors do you have? Check off any factors that apply:

☐ Preexisting health issues

☐ Gastrointestinal problems (e.g., irritable bowel syndrome, Crohn's disease, SIBO or Small Intestinal Bacterial Overgrowth)

☐ High stress, either personally or professionally

☐ A busy, on-the-go lifestyle

☐ Lack of exercise or a very sedentary lifestyle

☐ Disrupted sleep patterns (fewer than seven hours of sleep per night)

☐ A diet low in nutritional value (Standard American Diet)

☐ Inconsistent or nonexistent vitamin supplementation

☐ Low water intake (less than half your body weight in ounces daily)

☐ Recent major life events (e.g., death of a loved one, divorce, new job, household move)

If you answered yes to any of these factors, consider additional nutritional support or lifestyle adjustments where possible. If you have multiple factors, supplementation could hold the key to feeling like yourself again!

All of these elements can compromise our absorption of critical vitamins and minerals. It's important to do your research and determine what works best for you and your lifestyle. Be realistic rather than idealistic in your approach, and always consult with your health care provider before making significant changes.

Remember: achieving optimal health is a journey unique to each individual. By understanding your personal nutritional needs and the factors that influence them, you can make informed decisions to support your well-being at the cellular level.

MICRONUTRIENTS AND RESILIENCE: A PROMISING STUDY

An Austrian intervention study coordinated by Biogena sought to determine whether a 12-week regimen of specially combined nutrients could affect resilience stress levels and overall well-being in healthy adults experiencing increased occupational stress.

The results were impressive:

- Cellular resilience increased by 15.3%
- Overall well-being improved by 78.9%
- Stress perception decreased by 44.5%

This is compelling evidence for the value of nutritional support. By understanding our unique nutritional needs and addressing deficiencies proactively, we can unlock our body's natural healing potential and build a stronger foundation for long-term health.

DR. DANIEL'S STORY: REVITALIZING HEALTH IN THE GOLDEN YEARS

At 72, Dr. Daniel came to IV Lounge facing typical age-related challenges: low energy, fatigue, slow cognition, lack of stamina, dehydration, and poor sleep. As we age, our cells' ability to regenerate, produce energy, and function optimally declines, leading to these common symptoms.

As a doctor of alternative medicine, Dr. Daniel understood the benefits of hydration and supplementation. Initially, he was skeptical of IV therapy, which he dismissed as a fad. This perspective is common, even among health professionals. Despite his reservations, Dr. Daniel's desire to feel better outweighed his skepticism, and he gave it a try.

He began a regimen of weekly Immunity IVs, committing to a month-long trial. The transformation was remarkable. After just a couple of sessions, we noticed a significant change. Dr. Daniel was more alert during treatments, no longer dozing off as he had before. The tired, withdrawn look on his face gave way to a brighter, more youthful appearance. His skin looked fuller, with fewer lines. The dark circles under his eyes were gone. Even his demeanor, though always pleasant, seemed cheerier.

The most rewarding outcome was seeing Dr. Daniel regain his energy and zest for life. This renewed vitality allowed him to continue his life's work as a physician, a calling he cherished. Today, Dr. Daniel maintains his health with monthly nutritional support and hydration treatments, never missing an appointment.

Dr. Daniel's experience underscores a crucial point: living with vitality in our later years requires targeted cellular nutrition.

Whether through IV vitamin therapy or other methods, replenishing what declines with age is essential to maintain optimally functioning cells.

THE CRUCIAL ROLE OF SUPPLEMENTS IN MODERN LIFE

In today's world, we face unprecedented exposure to toxins and what some refer to as xenobiotics—the chemicals of our modern life. Our bodies are constantly battling EMFs, dirty electricity, water pollution, chemicals, and air pollution, among other environmental stressors discussed in the Chapter 4. If we don't address these disruptive elements, our need for supplemental nutrients becomes even more critical, because these toxins can interfere with vitamin and mineral absorption. The reality of daily toxin exposure also makes it challenging to trust that we're getting all the nutrients we need from food and water alone.

A common misconception persists that vitamin supplementation is unnecessary—that it's just "expensive urine" and we should simply eat the right foods. My response to this is simple: what is your health worth? Can you confidently rely on the quantity and quality of your daily diet, which varies based on the season and your lifestyle choices? Even if you consistently eat a plant-based diet of whole foods and non-GMO organic produce, you can still fall short of optimal nutrient levels. There's always room for improvement at the cellular level in today's health challenging world.

It's true that IV formulas contain water-soluble vitamins processed through the liver and kidneys, sometimes resulting in colorful urine. However, the cellular impact of these nutrients can last for days, weeks, or even months, depending on the cells affected. What may appear as "expensive urine" has already made a rapid and replenishing impact on your body's cells.

For perspective, consider that the lifespan of one vitamin infusion on the cells of the gastrointestinal tract can last several days, while impact on cells in other areas of the body last for months or even years. For example, B12 can be stored in the liver of a healthy person for 2-5 years, yet it is still a common deficiency. You may not be aware of what's happening at the cellular level, but you'll likely notice improvements in sleep quality, mood, energy levels, immune function, and skin appearance as your cellular health improves. Interestingly, many clients become more aware of their nutrient levels when they start to feel depleted, rather than when they're experiencing the full benefits of optimal nutrition.

Consistently feeding our cells with a diverse array of micronutrients boosts the production of healthy cells and enhances our resilience against illness and disease.

THE IMPORTANCE OF CONSISTENT NUTRIENT SUPPLEMENTATION

Just as regular exercise is crucial for physical fitness, consistent vitamin supplementation is essential for optimal health. Our nutrient needs fluctuate daily based on the factors we've discussed. Lifestyle choices, diet, stress levels, emotional state, toxin exposure, and preexisting health conditions all impact how our bodies absorb and use nutrients.

If you suspect that any of these factors might be affecting your nutrient absorption, it's wise to consult with your health care provider. You may need to adjust your supplementation routine to meet your body's changing needs.

Our bodies are remarkably intelligent, using the nutrients they require and excreting excess through the liver and kidneys. It's important to note that it's nearly impossible to overdose on water-soluble vitamins, which are typically used in vitamin infusions.

For generally healthy individuals who've been recently feeling depleted or "off", a nutrient deficiency could be the culprit. A practical way to determine if this is the case is to undergo a therapeutic trial of IV treatments over two to three weeks.

At IV Lounge, we typically recommend one IV session per week for two to four weeks, depending on your health history and individual circumstances. If you notice improvements in energy levels, mood, mental clarity, sleep quality, or overall wellness, it's likely that addressing nutrient deficiencies is key to helping you feel better.

However, if you don't experience any benefits after this trial period, other health conditions may be at play. In this case, it's advisable to seek further medical advice. It is important to consult with your primary care physician before starting any alternative therapy, especially if you're under medical care for other conditions.

While vitamin deficiencies are often easily correctable, leaving them unaddressed can lead to chronic symptoms, illness, and even disease. It's crucial to take a proactive approach to your nutritional health.

The government's guidelines for daily supplementation offer a one-size-fits-all approach, but they don't account for our individual uniqueness. Our nutrient needs can vary significantly from person to person and even day to day. We encourage you to research and identify the appropriate dosages for your specific health needs and lifestyle.

Regularly assess your vitamin needs based on the factors we've discussed. Think of it as setting a danger level for your health—are you at level 5 (optimal health) or level 1 (severe deficiency)? Adjust your supplementation strategy accordingly.

In terms of efficiency and effectiveness, intravenous vitamin therapy is a superior method of targeted cellular nutrition. However, if you're not comfortable with needles, sublingual vitamins from reputable sources can be a suitable alternative.

Remember, you have options for supporting your cellular health. By making informed choices about supplementation, you can maintain your desired lifestyle and live with enhanced vitality.

ACTIONS YOU CAN TAKE TODAY

1. **DISEASE OR DEFICIENCY**: Do your homework, sometimes symptoms are the body's cry for nutrients.
2. **QUALITY NOT QUANTITY**: Chose high-quality vitamins based on your needs, not your neighbors. The need is universal not the amount!
3. **OPTIMAL LEVELS, OPTIMAL LIFE**: Maintain adequate levels of nutrients every day. As the demands of life increase so does our need for essential vitamins.
4. **CONSISTENCY IS KEY**: Consistent nutrient levels are essential for optimal health. Lifestyles, stress and toxins can affect those levels daily.

By addressing toxicity and deficiency, we can take significant strides toward the goal of optimal health and vitality.

To help you succeed, I've designed something truly special—your personal set of Vitality Action Cards! These beautiful reminders (free PDF download) keep you focused on the practices that matter most. Place them anywhere you need inspiration. I'd love to see how they're helping you thrive—share a photo of your cards in their new home! Get your gifts now: www. thevitalitysolutionbook.com/gifts

"All chronic and degenerative diseases are caused by two and only two major problems—toxicity and deficiency."

—CHARLOTTE GERSON (AUTHOR, THE
GERSON THERAPY)

"Time and health are two precious assets that we don't recognize and appreciate until they have been depleted."

-Dennis Waitley

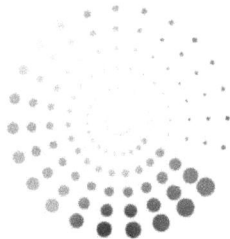

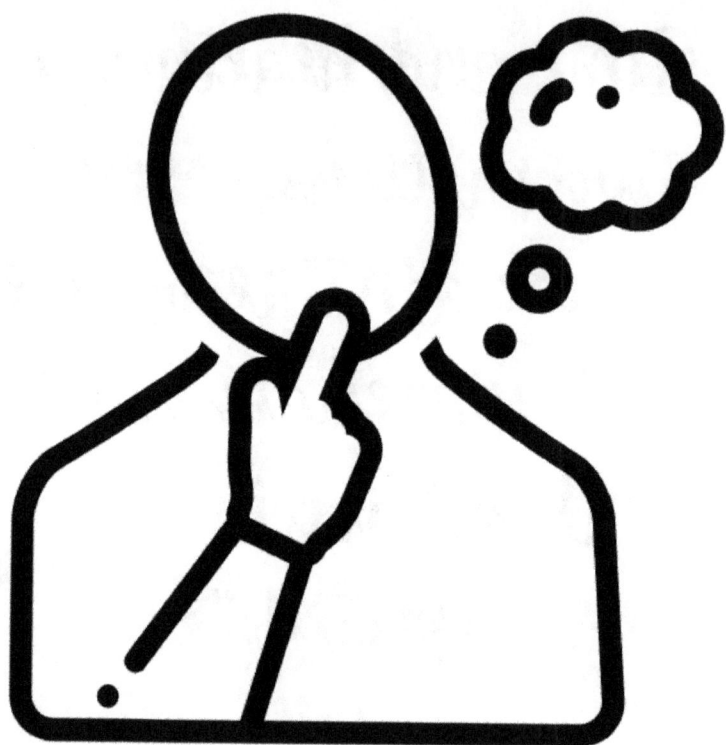

DISEASE OR
DEFFICIENCY?

#1

DO YOUR HOMEWORK, SOMETIMES SYMPTOMS CAN BE OUR BODY'S CRY FOR VITAMINS.

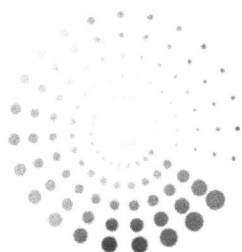

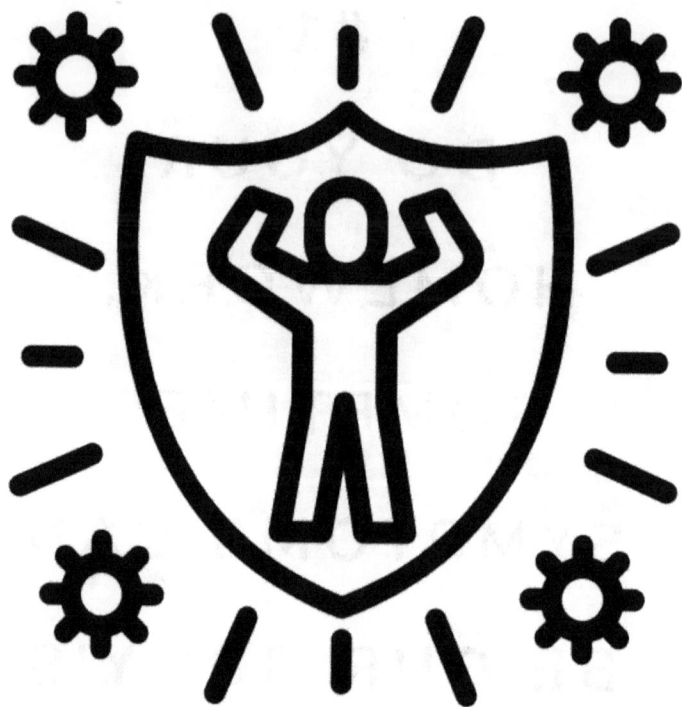

QUALITY NOT
QUANTITY

#2

CHOOSE HIGH QUALITY VITAMINS BASED ON WHAT YOUR BODY NEEDS, NOT YOUR NEIGHBORS

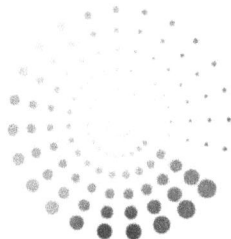

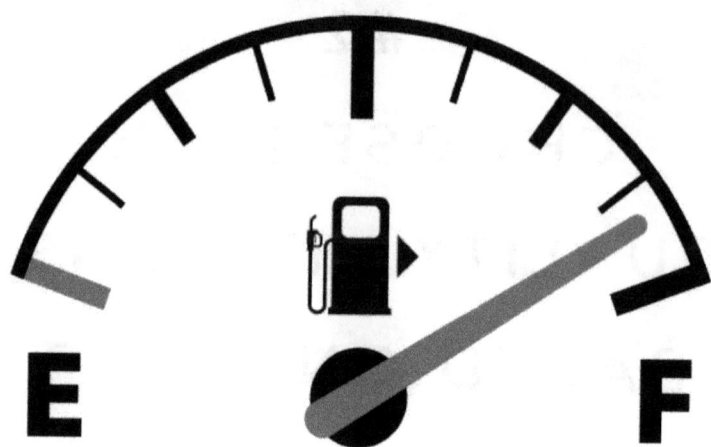

OPTIMAL LEVELS
OPTIMIZE LIFE

#3
MAINTAIN ADEQUATE LEVELS OF NUTRIENTS EVERY DAY.

AS THE DEMANDS OF LIFE INCREASE SO DOES THE BODIES NEED FOR NUTRITION

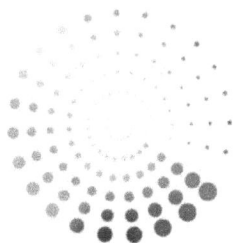

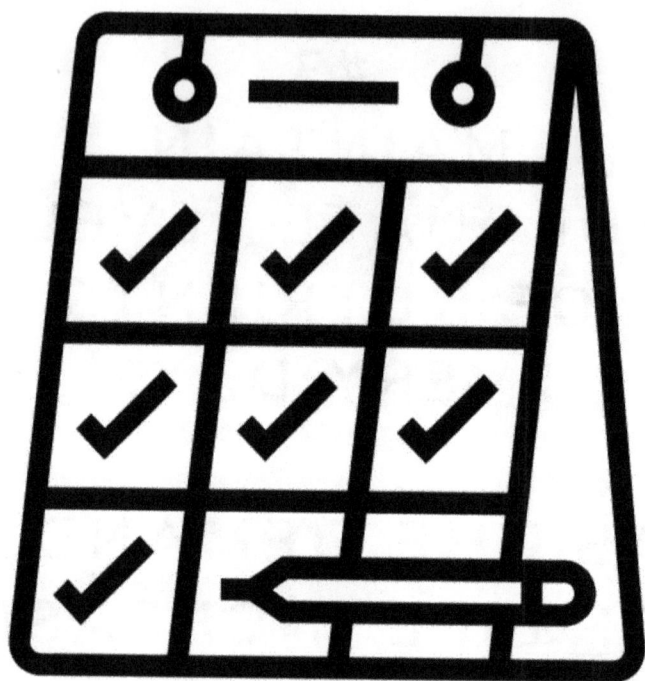

CONSISTENCY
IS KEY

#4

REGULAR SUPPLEMENTATION IS ESSENTIAL FOR OPTIMAL HEALTH.

TOXINS, DAILY STRESS & LIFE CAN DEPLETE US OF VITAL NUTRIENT RESERVES.

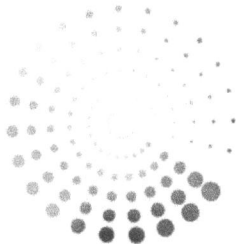

longevity

BIOHACKING HEALTH AND VITALITY

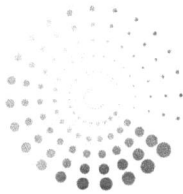

"You can't help getting older, but you don't have to get old."

—GEORGE BURNS

The meaning of longevity is "long life." While some argue that lifespan matters more than life quality, I strongly disagree. Recently, during an IV treatment session, one of my regular clients in his early 80s put it perfectly, "What's the point in living longer if your quality of life is bad?"

In this chapter, I want to explore powerful but often overlooked approaches to healing and longevity that are gaining recognition in scientific circles. We'll examine how our cellular health depends on what we feed our bodies, and how we can optimize our cells' function naturally. We'll look at how lifestyle choices impact longevity, and how our mindset about aging—whether positive or negative—can influence our cellular resilience. The exciting news is that the tools for "biohacking" our cellular longevity exist today and are waiting to be used!

I'll share some remarkable experiences that transformed my own health and vitality. I'll also tell a very personal story that I rarely share: my experience of being old before my time and how it affected my family. This experience now fuels my passion to help others take control of their health destiny.

QUALITY VS. QUANTITY

Until recently, living vibrantly into our 90s or even 100s seemed impossible—we focused on extending life without considering its quality. But advances in longevity science have revealed both what makes our cells age *and* how we might slow or counteract this process to a greater degree. As someone fascinated by human biology and cellular healing, I've studied this field for decades. The exciting truth is that we can choose to live our golden years with vitality—it's within our grasp!

Who wants to reach one hundred if they're immobile, cognitively impaired, and dependent on others? Many of us assume we'll follow our grandparents' path: gradually losing abilities until we return to a childlike state. But this isn't inevitable. I know because I've lived both possibilities.

Near the end of my illness, I received what I now see as a blessing: a glimpse of what awaited me in my old age if I changed nothing. Though this story is painful to share, I tell it because it demonstrates how divine intervention and personal choice can transform our health trajectory. It's rare to get a preview of our future with the chance or ability to change it.

MY "ELDERLY" STORY

In my 40s, after years of health struggles, I experienced what I can only describe as premature aging, both physically and mentally. I view this experience as both a blessing and a curse. It was a stark preview of what I wanted to avoid in my actual golden years, and, thankfully, it is a story I can now tell in the past tense.

My health journey was long and challenging. I went from one medical institution to another, seeing every type of specialist and enduring countless tests—some so difficult they left me with PTSD. Despite spending hundreds of thousands of dollars searching for answers, or even a doctor who would truly listen, I found no solutions.

After eighteen months of aggressive Lyme treatments, my quality of life vanished as my muscle function deteriorated. I became dependent on others for basic daily tasks and getting my children where they needed to be. My mitochondria—the cellular energy factories that generate adenosine triphosphate (ATP)—were severely depleted. Simple movements, breathing, or even laughing would trigger seizures. (Who knew laughter took so much energy?) I went from using a cane to a walker and, finally, a wheelchair. As my muscles failed, I needed oxygen support since every breath consumed precious energy I needed just to survive. Even swallowing became difficult, and choking and gagging became frighteningly common.

The seizures from my failing muscles made it nearly impossible to speak coherently or find words, partly due to the oxygen deprivation affecting my brain. Simple tasks like showering and doing laundry could trigger muscle seizures and garbled speech, and painful muscle spasms or choking episodes that often led to emergency room visits.

As a type A personality, I prided myself on maintaining appearances during those years, but truthfully, I survived only through divine intervention and my amazing support network of girlfriends. Few people besides my boys, family and closest friends ever witnessed the seizures or heard my struggling speech —I just kept smiling and pretending. I rarely allowed people to take photos of me in the wheelchair or using oxygen, and it's something I regret because it now appears that during those years I didn't exist.

Near what we thought might be the end, even tiny efforts resulted in seizures and unintelligible speech. I was essentially living in an elderly body decades too soon. I was dependent on others, in cognitive decline, and unable to manage basic needs. The hardest part was watching my family's anguish over my condition. It was the only time I considered that my death might be easier on them than watching me suffer. As a person of faith, I knew God had a purpose for this suffering. He had already used my situation to inspire others and share my faith, even when I felt useless. I've always believed every circumstance has a purpose, and God carried me through my weakest moments.

By God's grace I survived, and I can now write about this time as a memory rather than my present reality. Each morning that I wake up breathing independently and walking on my own fills me with immense gratitude. My conversations with God throughout this journey could fill another book, but I knew this second chance at life demanded action. As soon as I was able, I committed to making IV therapy accessible to others and sharing what I'd learned.

Creating awareness about alternative health tools empowers people and offers hope. We have the power to write our own health story—choosing either a life full of vitality or one of helplessness. As you continue reading, you'll understand the control you have over your health, without needing to spend your savings like I did.

GOOD GENES ARE NO GUARANTEE

The debate continues about genetics versus lifestyle in determining longevity. Some believe genetics dictate lifespan, while others emphasize lifestyle choices. But does having centenarian grandparents guarantee longevity despite poor diet and lifestyle choices? My research and personal experience suggest otherwise.

As previous chapters showed, our cellular health responds to diet and lifestyle choices. A family history of longevity doesn't give us license to eat poorly and remain sedentary. The cause-and-effect relationship is clear and significant.

According to Dr. Joe Dispenza, even our body's energy field, both internal and external, can transform cellular behavior. When we nourish our cells with proper fuel, energy, and a positive environment, we influence our lifespan.

True longevity isn't just about time—it's about maintaining full functionality of mind, body and soul until your final day, hopefully with a smile! To achieve this, we must perform five key tasks in sequence:

1. Make health the priority-(Mindset)
2. Build a healthy foundation (Immunity)

3. Clean house (Detox)
4. Strengthen reserves (Restoration)
5. Revitalize and optimize cells (Longevity)

By developing healthier, more resilient cellular structures, we can slow aging and protect against illness and disease.

FUEL FOR OUR CELLS

If we want our cells to function optimally, we need to consider what we're feeding them.

I hate to say it, but you really are what you eat! As a food lover who enjoys wine, chocolate and a fancy meal every so often, I understand the struggle. My willpower around food, especially in the winter, has often resembled that of a bear just coming out of hibernation. But recently, I've experienced firsthand how viewing food as cellular fuel, rather than just calories, can transform health. After years of worrying about being alive, I can now focus on living my life optimally fueled.

Growing up, my mom was always reading books. Though she was never afforded the opportunity to get a college education, she was wiser than most college-educated people and proactively studied the ins and outs of healthy living. She was at the forefront of the alternative health movement before it became mainstream.

Perhaps not surprisingly, then, I raised my boys on the mantra, "If you put junk in, you'll get junk out!" I emphasized that fueling your body with junk is a guarantee your body and brain will not perform to the best of their ability.

Even before my health crisis, before I deeply understood nutrition, I knew the basics. I knew saturated fats were harmful, too much salt was disastrous, and fried foods were the worst. I knew sugar created intense highs followed by crashing lows. Looking back now, though, I laugh. If I'd known then what I know now, I would have avoided those drive-thru meals on busy days, weekly pizzas, and constant caffeine fixes.

Food is fuel, plain and simple. It keeps our motors running.

If you eat unhealthy food, you'll feel unhealthy. Empty calories lead to weight gain without providing real energy for your cells. You'll experience headaches, mood swings, acne, fatigue, cognitive issues, and other unpleasant symptoms. It's unavoidable.

If you've spent years eating a diet high in sugar, saturated fat, daily meat, or frequent fast food, you might not notice these effects because your body has adapted to running on empty. While our bodies are remarkably adaptable, this tolerance is temporary. As cells age, they become less forgiving of poor fuel choices, and the results are conditions like high blood pressure, diabetes, autoimmune disorders, and even mental health issues.

Just as Rome wasn't built in a day, transitioning to healthy eating takes time. I don't recommend switching to a whole-foods, plant-based diet overnight unless you're prepared for bathroom emergencies. The high fiber content, while essential, can have a powerful effect on unprepared digestive systems.

This adjustment period might also discourage some people, as your body often goes through a detox phase when you start eating healthier. But don't worry—these responses are positive signs, even if they're uncomfortable. When your cells receive better fuel, they begin to purge long-stored toxins. While not always pleasant, this cleansing process is worth the temporary discomfort.

Important facts about digestion:

- Food typically takes three days to move through your digestive system
- Breaking sugar, carb and salt cravings requires three weeks of healthy eating
- Digestion uses 10 to 15% of your daily energy
- Plant-based meals digest in about 24 hours
- Standard American Diet meals take up to three days to digest, wasting valuable energy

Here's an interesting fact: taste buds renew every 10 to 14 days, not every seven years. This constant renewal helps maintain our sense of taste and explains why you can retrain your palate to enjoy healthier foods.

Do you have any of the following issues:

☐ inflammation

☐ pain

☐ low energy

☐ anxiety

☐ mood swings

☐ sugar/salt cravings

☐ insomnia

What if you could resolve these issues naturally, without medication, and at minimal cost? It's possible when we give our bodies proper fuel.

Our food choices are crucial to longevity and symptom-free living. What we eat becomes fuel for our cells, laying the foundation for either health or disease. Healthy eating is not about diet it is about FUEL plain and simple.

I have witnessed and experienced the dramatic difference between using the right and wrong nutritional fuel. After years of poor food choices and ingrained habits, changing your lifestyle isn't easy. Sometimes it takes dramatic measures to reset those pleasure receptors and break habitual patterns.

FASTING

"The best of all medicines are resting and fasting."

—Benjamin Franklin

This is where fasting can make a difference. While fasting might sound extreme, it has helped thousands of people extend their lifespan and eliminate medications, steering them away from disease. I'm one of those people. Though I struggle with food like anyone else and live an active lifestyle, my desire to live pain-free, to maintain a healthy body, and to avoid premature death now outweighs my old habits.

Truthfully, it took my dangerously poor lab results—even after my near-death experience—to motivate me to make real change. Fasting helped break my unhealthy eating cycles and allowed me to transition more easily to a whole-food, plant-based lifestyle.

As I write this, I'm completing my second water-only fast at True North Health clinic in Santa Rosa, California. My first fast there lasted 12 days, and it taught me what I could handle mentally and physically. The results were so positive that my doctor recommended I repeat this fast every six months to address multiple long-standing health issues from my chronic illness.

During this second fast, I managed 16 days on water alone, successfully addressing another layer of health challenges. I've lost stubborn weight that persisted despite regular exercise and a whole-foods diet (though stress, hormones, and age didn't help). While fasting isn't a weight-loss solution—you'll regain some weight—it can reset your metabolism and fundamentally change your eating habits.

I mention this because many Americans fuel themselves with the Standard American Diet (SAD), which promotes disease alongside poor lifestyle choices. The SAD way of living means you are eating highly processed pesticide-laden food, full of excess sugar, high calorie but low in nutrient density. It is also high in saturated and trans fats (cholesterol makers), high in additives and preservatives that our immune system considers "foreign invaders" and in an attempt to get rid of these "unknowns" unleashes a systemic inflammatory response which is the root cause of many health maladies and diseases in America today. This type of diet also leads to numerous digestive issues, mood and brain function problems, not to mention the weight gain and creation of toxins which go hand in hand because fat cells make great hiding places for toxins!

Pharmaceutical companies make billions from chronic illnesses triggered by the Standard American Diet (SAD). This growing trend should alarm us all and serve as a wake-up call. Let's fix what we can while we can!

While fasting might seem trendy, it's an ancient practice that dates back to biblical times and remains important in many religions.

In ancient Greece, Hippocrates prescribed fasting for infections and acute illnesses. Many world religions still advocate fasting periods, recognizing both its mental and physical benefits.

Biblical fasting served multiple purposes: clarity, spiritual connection, mourning and worship: "I ate no delicacies, no meat or wine entered my mouth, nor did I anoint myself at all, for the full three weeks" (*Daniel 10:3 ESV*); "So, he was there with the Lord forty days and forty nights. He neither ate bread nor drank water. And he wrote on the tablets the words of the covenant, the Ten Commandments" (*Exodus 34:28 ESV*).

Both the Old and New Testaments emphasize fasting—abstaining from food or drink to focus on prayer and seek God's will. Scripture mentions fasting more than 70 times. As a person of faith, I'm surprised I didn't consider fasting sooner, but God's timing is always perfect.

Today's approaches range from intermittent fasting to multi-day fasts. Short-term or intermittent fasting is accessible—it's free, requires no memberships, equipment, or expensive supplements. These shorter fasts can easily fit into busy schedules. If you have health issues, fasts longer than 24 hours should be medically supervised at facilities like True North in Santa Rosa.

Intermittent fasting involves adjusting your eating window—you don't even need to change your diet. This was my gateway into fasting, thanks to my eldest son Nick, a certified personal trainer and lifelong student of nutrition. In an effort to clean up his own diet, deal with work stress as a construction superintendent, and support his busy schedule, he turned to intermittent fasting. He achieved stellar results with little effort. When I saw his success, I thought, "I could reduce my eating window. Why not?!"

I bought Dr. Mindy Pelz's book *Fast Like a Girl* and began my experimentation with intermittent fasting.

STEM CELLS AND FASTING

Stem cells are the foundation of every organ and tissue in our body. These remarkable cells can both reproduce and generate newer, healthier cells, giving them a crucial role in healing damaged or diseased organs.

Fasting—whether periodic, intermittent, or prolonged—triggers stem cell–dependent regeneration in the immune system, nervous system and pancreas. During fasting, the body undergoes autophagy ("self-eating"), where damaged or "rogue" cells are consumed and replaced by healthier cells through stem cell activation. Cellular apoptosis also occurs and results in the orderly death of bad cells.

According to Dr. Mindy Pelz, here's what happens in your body during different fasting periods:

13 to 15 hours:

- Human growth hormone (HGH) increases
- Inflammation reduces
- Fat burning begins

- Ketones increase
- Energy and focus improve

17 hours:

- Cellular detoxification activates
- Cellular repair begins
- Immune function improves

24 hours:

- Intestinal stem cells regenerate
- Gamma-aminobutyric acid (GABA) production increases
- Brain healing begins
- Autoimmune healing starts

36 hours:

- Glucose stores reduce
- Insulin levels drop
- Fat burning increases
- Detoxification deepens
- Anti-aging processes activate

48 hours:

- Dopamine receptors reset
- Anxiety and depression reduce (through increased GABA)
- Antioxidant production rises
- HGH increases by 500%

72 hours:

- Autophagy peaks
- Immune stem cell production maximizes
- Musculoskeletal stem cells generate
- Healing accelerates

Three-day fast: At this point, autophagy peaks. Your healthy cells begin consuming damaged or abnormal cells, including some cancer cells (depending on their stage). These problematic cells are often the result of toxin exposure, inflammation or genetic mutations. And another process called apoptosis activates, triggering the programmed death of unnecessary or abnormal cells.

Your body enters ketosis, burning fat instead of sugar for fuel. Since only healthy cells can effectively use fat for fuel, problematic cells become targets for autophagy or apoptosis. Your immune system undergoes significant repair as harmful cells decrease, accelerating healing. Your body, which is now spending minimal energy on digestion, focuses instead on healing.

One-week fast: Beyond three days, healing intensifies at the cellular level. This extraordinary phase features sustained autophagy and increased stem cell production. The healing effects continue for months after the fast ends.

Healing rates vary by individual and condition. Think of it like peeling an onion: each layer of cellular dysfunction you remove reduces the toxic burden on your body and the energy consumed by illness or disease.

FASTING MYTHS DEBUNKED

Myth: *Fasting destroys muscle mass.*

Truth: Your body won't break down muscle until your body fat drops below 4%. Even elite marathon runners maintain around 8% body fat. During fasting, your body preserves muscle and releases human growth hormone (HGH), supporting lean muscle mass. Any muscle deflation that occurs during fasting is typically water loss that returns with rehydration.

Myth: *Fasting causes low blood sugar.*

Truth: While you might experience initial symptoms like shakiness or lightheadedness when you start fasting, these usually pass. However, if you're prone to hypoglycemia or consume lots of sugar or starch, consult your physician first. Once your body becomes "fat-adapted," it will efficiently use fat instead of sugar for fuel.

Myth: *Fasting causes nutrient deficiencies.*

Truth: Fasting helps conserve nutrients. Your body reduces vitamin and mineral excretion during fasting. With fewer bowel movements, you lose fewer nutrients. Most people maintain stable levels of electrolytes, magnesium, potassium, calcium and phosphorus during extended fasts. However, if you're already nutrient deficient, longer fasts should be medically supervised.

MY INTRODUCTION TO FASTING

In February 2024, I had regular lab work done to monitor my ongoing health challenges: autoimmune thyroiditis, hepatitis, chronic Epstein Barr infections, and other conditions that required constant attention.

I hadn't been feeling well. I was struggling with stress and poor dietary choices from working long hours. My adrenals were in overdrive from circumstances beyond my control. When we ran the labs, I expected poor results but wasn't prepared for how serious things had become.

The results were alarming, far outside normal ranges. My condition demanded immediate intervention, either through medication and lifestyle changes or something more dramatic, to prevent a stroke or heart attack.

I tried cleaning up my paleo diet first—eliminating alcohol and sugar and adding more vegetables. I was already exercising regularly, and I increased my meditative prayer practice and added "grounding" breaks to lower my cortisol levels. Despite adding adrenal supplements to support my stressed organs, nothing seemed to help. My weight kept climbing from high cortisol, and inflammation overwhelmed my body.

At this critical point, realizing I couldn't help others if I couldn't help myself. Dr. Dang, my friend and colleague, suggested water-only fasting at True North Medical Clinic in Santa Rosa, California. Her colleague had interned there and witnessed remarkable recoveries through fasting.

Preferring natural treatments, I refused medication despite the severity of my situation. I committed to a two-week program while my husband signed up for five days to address his own lab numbers and stress. After initial consultations, we were cleared to begin.

During my initial clinic assessment, the doctor determined I wasn't healthy enough for immediate water-only fasting. He started me with a four-day juice fast while monitoring my bloodwork. This gentler approach proved wise—by day five, my labs improved enough to begin water-only fasting. My husband completed his five-day fast successfully, though with less enthusiasm than me! His 60-day follow-up labs showed significant improvements, helping reverse what could have become irreversible damage.

While I was excited about fasting, I won't pretend it was easy. Healing involved many physical and mental challenges, but the results proved worth every difficult moment. My body allowed me to fast for 12 full days, detoxifying and repairing itself. I lost 23 pounds, and though some weight returned, the crushing burden of inflammation lifted. For the first time in years, I felt like myself again. Even my doctor, initially skeptical, expressed amazement at my progress.

Three months later, my lab results were remarkable—my numbers had dropped by half. Though some issues remain works in progress, this represents a massive victory. The doctor explained that my complex health situation would require several fasting treatments to address multiple layers of dysfunction. As someone repeatedly told there was no hope for recovery, I'll gladly return for more treatments to maintain this vital, pain-free life.

When I returned home, my relationship with food had transformed. I couldn't believe how much better I felt, and it was then that I realized how much pain I'd been living with daily. Now, I primarily eat plant-based whole foods. I limit salt and meat and avoid sugar, dairy, and unhealthy oils. My energy levels are higher than they've been in years. I scheduled my second water-only fast at True North a few months later, July 2024 as mentioned earlier.

The concept of drinking only water for days or weeks might seem illogical, and many think I'm crazy. But I tell skeptical friends and family that if they could feel the difference between my previous constant pain and my current well-being, they'd understand my motivation to fast.

> *"Fasting is a window into the extraordinary power we all possess, the body's ability to heal itself!"*
>
> —CAREY MENCARINI

LIFESTYLE

Our daily habits speak volumes about our health priorities without saying a word. How we live reveals our values, beliefs, and the priority we place on our health. The centenarians living in the "Blue Zones" (these are geographical regions where people have been found to live longer, healthier lives than most, often reaching 100) demonstrate this—they prioritize health through consistent daily practices. Their habits have become a blueprint for longevity. Here are seven key principles shared among these long-lived communities:

1. **MOVE**: The world's healthiest centenarians don't rely on gyms or marathons—they move naturally throughout their day, multiple times daily.
2. **PURPOSE**: Everyone needs to feel needed. Having a clear purpose provides motivation to stay healthy and engaged.

3. **UNPLUG**: They make time to disconnect a couple of times each day, allowing for restoration and renewal.
4. **PLANT-BASED DIET**: They focus on natural foods provided by nature, not processed products.
5. **RELATIONSHIPS**: They prioritize meaningful connections and make time to nurture them.
6. **POSITIVE MINDSET**: They nurture a positive mindset.
7. **COMMUNITY**: They maintain strong connections with like-minded people through community involvement.

Beyond these seven principles, there are three other key lifestyle factors impact our cellular function:

1. Sleep
2. Stress
3. Environment

Let's look at each of these in turn.

Sleep

Poor sleep patterns suppress our immune system, leaving us vulnerable to illness and disease. Quality sleep allows our immune system to enter repair mode—without it, we miss this crucial natural "reboot" time.

Stress

While we all know stress is harmful, we often let it control our lives until illness forces us to pay attention. Learning stress management techniques and using appropriate supplements can boost cellular longevity and health.

Exercise

With exercise, the goal isn't perfection or athletic achievement—it's simply moving your body to benefit your cells. Walking for just fifteen minutes improves blood circulation, opens lymphatic valves (which only activate through movement), and increases oxygen flow to the brain for clearer thinking. Movement also triggers endorphin release, improving mood and motivation. This simple activity enhances cellular communication throughout your body.

Environment

Location matters, but it shouldn't determine your health! City dwellers face more environmental toxins than those in rural areas, who have access to fresher air and cleaner water. According to Environmental Working Group studies, increased air pollution raises risks of:

- Stroke
- Heart disease
- Lung cancer
- Chronic respiratory diseases
- Asthma

Research also suggests that air pollution may contribute to obesity by discouraging outdoor exercise. Many water sources contain questionable chemicals that can impact health.

However, we're not helpless against environmental challenges. As discussed in Chapter 4, we can mitigate these exposures through regular detoxification practices regardless of where you live. We have the power to enhance our cellular function through daily choices that promote health and vitality.

PERCEPTION IS EVERYTHING: IS THE GLASS HALF-FULL OR HALF-EMPTY?

How do you view your "golden years"? Will you embrace them, or do they fill you with dread? Our perception of aging powerfully influences our reality. If we see aging negatively, that fear manifests in our bodies at the cellular level. A single negative thought can trigger a cascade of cellular events, creating a chain reaction of negative responses.

When you think a thought, your brain releases neurotransmitters —chemical messengers that communicate with your nervous system and brain. These neurotransmitters influence cells throughout your body. Positive thoughts can protect neurons and create lasting benefits, while negative thoughts can damage our cells.

According to researchers at the University of California San Francisco, a positive mindset can actually *reverse* the aging process. It's not just your chronological age that matters, but how you feel about aging. If we all understood how our thoughts influence our health, wouldn't we all try to maintain a more positive outlook?

Remember René Descartes' famous phrase, "I think therefore I am"? We are what we eat *and* what we think—both shape who we become, become, how we live our lives, and our longevity.

In the United States today, life expectancy averages 79 years—a dramatic increase from a century ago, when it was 54. Dr. Marie Bernard, deputy director of NIH's National Institute on Aging, has noted, "Now if you make it to age 65, the likelihood that you'll make it to 85 is very high. And if you make it to 85, the likelihood that you'll make it to 92 is very high. People are living longer, and it's happening across the globe."

The World Health Organization reports:

- Global aging is happening faster than ever before
- As of 2020, people over 60 outnumbered children under 5
- Between 2015 and 2050, the over-60 population will nearly double from 12% to 22%
- By 2050, the number of people 80+ will triple to 426 million

And here are a few more fascinating facts about aging:

- Globally, Japanese people have the longest, healthiest lives.
- In 195 of 198 countries, women outlive men, by an average of six extra years.
- Southern Africa has the shortest life expectancies in the world.
- New research suggests humans that could potentially live to 150 years of age.

BIOHACKING OUR CELLS: CELLULAR LANDSCAPING

We've built a foundation for cellular vitality through strengthening immunity, removing toxins, and restoring nutrients. Let's take the next step: reinforcing our cellular fortress with energetic cells that promote vibrant longevity.

I'll share simple but effective anti-aging biohacks that I use regularly and are available to everyone. We've discussed fasting to generate new stem cells crucial for immunity, disease resistance, and longevity. We understand how diet and lifestyle choices affect cellular integrity. Now let's explore additional accessible ways to strengthen your cellular warehouse.

NAD (Nicotinamide Adenine Dinucleotide):

Often called the "Fountain of Youth," this remarkable coenzyme is essential for cellular metabolism, DNA repair, and neuroprotection. Scientists believe it can actually reverse aging and age-related diseases. At IV Lounge, I've witnessed its game-changing effects personally and through countless client experiences with NAD IVs and injections.

While all vitamins serve important cellular functions, NAD uniquely powers every cell in the body. For those over 50, like myself, NAD production naturally decreases with age, making supplementation crucial for maintaining quality of life and slowing the aging process of our cells.

Consider all the benefits of NAD IV supplementation:

- Enhances collagen production
- Reduces premature aging signs

- Improves mental clarity and memory
- Protects brain cells
- Boosts energy and metabolism
- Enhances exercise performance
- Reduces muscle recovery time and pain
- Improves insulin sensitivity
- Increases stamina and drive
- Enhances sun damage protection
- Supports weight management
- Strengthens immune function
- Promotes restorative sleep
- Slows the overall effects of aging

Symptoms of low NAD include:

- Accelerated aging
- Fatigue
- Declining brain function
- Increased risk of age-related diseases (Alzheimer's, dementia)
- Sun sensitivity
- Weight gain
- Muscle weakness
- Decreased skin elasticity
- Wrinkles, and
- Reduced stamina.

PEMF (Pulsed Electro-Magnetic Frequency):

PEMF therapy revitalizes damaged cells using low-intensity emissions that mirror the natural frequencies of the brain, heart, and other vital organs. These carefully calibrated waveforms energize our cellular batteries (mitochondria), increasing cellular voltage, boosting ATP production, and eliminating toxic free radicals.

Energized cells better absorb nutrients, which accelerates healing and boosts immunity against various infections.

Our planet naturally produces electromagnetic and vibratory frequencies, and our bodies operate on a similar electromagnetic energy. However, we are now surrounded by artificial EMF radiation and "dirty electricity," which interferes with normal cell function and can lead to:

- Chronic stress
- Free radical damage
- Oxidative stress
- Chronic inflammation
- Calcium leaching from bones
- Excessive calcium in the cells According to EMF expert Lloyd Burrell, author of *Electric Sense*, daily EMF exposure can cause:
- DNA damage
- Blood-brain barrier leakage
- Leaky gut
- Fertility issues
- Various cancers
- Sleep disorders
- Heart disease
- Neurological disease

These symptoms suggest that disrupted electromagnetic frequencies and cellular de-energizing might contribute to disease, aging, and immune system breakdown—and they help explain PEMF therapy's remarkable results.

Healing requires cellular energy, which PEMF therapy provides while promoting the parasympathetic state necessary for healing. A child's cells typically maintain 90 millivolts, enabling faster healing, nutrient absorption, and toxin elimination. As we age, cellular voltage decreases, accelerating aging and our vulnerability to disease. PEMF therapy can restore youthful cellular voltage levels.

My PEMF Journey

Early in my health struggles, I developed rheumatoid arthritis and fibromyalgia syndrome, which caused swollen joints and full-body muscle pain. As a busy mother managing my boys' packed sports and school schedules, I desperately needed relief that neither diet nor medication provided. Despite trying numerous therapies—supplements, meditation, yoga, biofeedback, acupuncture—nothing provided adequate relief.

Sleep-deprived from pain and constantly sick due to my compromised immunity, I reluctantly turned to narcotics. This only created new problems. But through a friend's connection, I learned about a child who had recovered from chronic illness using a PEMF mat.

Willing to try anything, I invested in a PEMF mat and used it three times daily for 30 minutes. Within a week, my pain had decreased; within a month, I had stopped all pain medications. The mat has become indispensable—I never travel without it and still use it daily. For those who can afford it, I highly recommend PEMF therapy as a versatile healing tool.

Red Light Therapy—Photo-biomodulation (PBM)

The sun emits various light wavelengths, including red and near-infrared light. These wavelengths are "bioactive" in humans, which means they affect the function of every cell in our bodies.

This versatile therapy offers multiple intensity levels and applications, addressing everything from immune function and inflammation to skin conditions. It supports pre- and post-surgical healing, enhances exercise performance, and provides anti-aging benefits.

Red light therapy works by enhancing cellular energy while reducing oxidative stress, thus improving blood flow. Research shows it also stimulates stem cell production.

Red light therapy

- Reduces inflammation
- Boosts collagen production, minimizing fine lines
- Increases energy, mood and stamina
- Enhances athletic performance and recovery
- Improves circulation
- Stimulates hair growth
- Strengthens immunity
- Reduces pain and scarring
- Boosts metabolism
- Improves skin texture and appearance

Client Story: Rob (Alopecia)

Rob Linson, a physical therapist familiar with alternative medicine, came to IV Lounge seeking hair growth solutions. He'd tried red light therapy elsewhere with disappointing results, noting that their equipment used different light colors and operated at a lower intensity, while their sessions were only 10 minutes compared to our 20-minute treatments.

Our Vitality Booth combines red and near-infrared light: the deepest-penetrating safe light wavelengths available. After about eleven sessions, Rob noticed new hair growth. He's thrilled with his progress and continues treatment. His experience shows how proper light therapy can offer noninvasive alternatives to surgery or pharmaceuticals, avoiding potential side effects. About his experience with IV Lounge, Rob remarked, "When you are a trailblazer, figuring out these medical issues on your own, there can be many missteps, but that does not mean the answer is not out there! ... I plan to continue doing regular red light therapy for general wellness."

My Story

I utilize various light therapy tools, including our Vitality Booth at IV Lounge, which combines red light with halotherapy (salt therapy).

I also own a class 3b medical-grade red light laser, which offers concentrated treatment of the following:

- Soft tissue injuries
- Surgical scars
- Wound healing
- Collagen stimulation
- Arthritic pain
- Cartilage repair

My Son's Success Story

My youngest son, Austin, was an aggressive high school basketball player who frequently needed healing from injuries. During one tournament, he severely sprained his ankle. Combining traditional RICE (rest, ice, compression, elevation) methods with laser treatment, he returned to play within three days, protected by a brace but virtually pain-free and without reinjury.

I consider a personal laser an essential health tool in my arsenal. I started with a Class 2 laser (around $2,000)—less powerful but still effective—before upgrading to my Class 3b medical-grade laser (aka-more power).

Photo-biomodulation, is the therapeutic technique in which specific wavelengths of light are used to stimulate cellular processes. This type of therapeutic technique has advanced remarkably in modern medicine. I hope more health care providers will incorporate this powerful healing modality to make it more widely accessible to everyone.

For those interested in cutting-edge developments, I recommend doing your own research on epigenetics, regenerative medicine, and companies like Biosplice that are pushing beyond the realm of anti-aging and into the realm of de-aging. The science of cellular renewal and resilience has progressed remarkably, offering exciting possibilities for health and longevity.

"It always seems impossible until it's done."

—NELSON MANDELA

SAMMY'S STORY: ONE PRO-BOXER'S PATH TO PEAK PERFORMANCE

Sammy came to IV Lounge seeking enhanced immunity and muscle function support during her intense boxing training. While she was preparing for nationals, she tried our NAD+ 100 IV before sparring. It was her first experience with IV therapy. During the peaceful infusion time, she appreciated the rest, and she noted improved hydration and stamina the following day.

After winning her sparring match, Sammy reported superior muscle performance and faster recovery. Encouraged, she increased to our maximum 250-milligram dose of NAD+ IV just before the World Title. The results were remarkable—she breezed through the exhausting "cutting" phase, then dominated her ten-round championship fight. While her opponent showed fatigue, Sammy maintained extraordinary energy and agility throughout, ultimately defeating the top-ranked contender.

Sammy is now a regular at IV Lounge, and her vibrant personality and beautiful spirit have made her a staff favorite. She continues to win titles and rise through the professional boxing ranks with grace. She feels grateful for the nutritional support and hydration that complement her demanding career. As a bright light and local hero, she inspires our community, and we're honored to support her success.

EMBRACING LONGEVITY WITH VITALITY

True longevity isn't just about extending life—it's about maintaining vibrant health throughout our years. Our cells form the foundation of this vitality, but they can only perform at their peak when given proper tools and support.

The good news? Many powerful changes require no financial investment:

- Shift your mindset about aging
- Choose nutrient-rich whole foods
- Practice stress management
- Prioritize quality sleep
- Move your body regularly
- Connect with community
- Maintain a positive outlook

For those ready to explore further, targeted interventions like fasting, IV therapy, PEMF, and red light therapy can enhance cellular health and accelerate results. Whatever path you choose, remember that small, consistent changes create lasting impact.

ACTIONS YOU CAN TAKE TODAY FOR OPTIMAL LONGEVITY

1. **AGING WELL:** Your mind decides your fate when it comes to aging gracefully. Why not embrace it with a healthy outlook?
2. **NO GUARANTEES:** Diet and lifestyle choices drive our cellular function or dysfunction, not our genes.
3. **QUALITY FUEL:** Quality foods create quality fuel for our cells to function properly. Junk in equals junk out!
4. **FIND BALANCE:** Focus on living a lifestyle that supports less stress, quality sleep, exercise and positivity.
5. **CELLULAR LONGEVITY:** Optimize your cellular resilience with various forms of biohacking.

"Pay your farmer, not your pharmacist."

—KELLY LÉVÊQUE

"you can't help
getting older.
but you don't have
to get old."

Karen Salmansohn

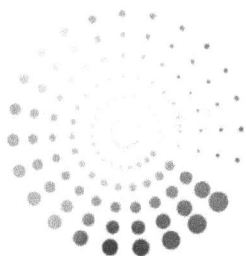

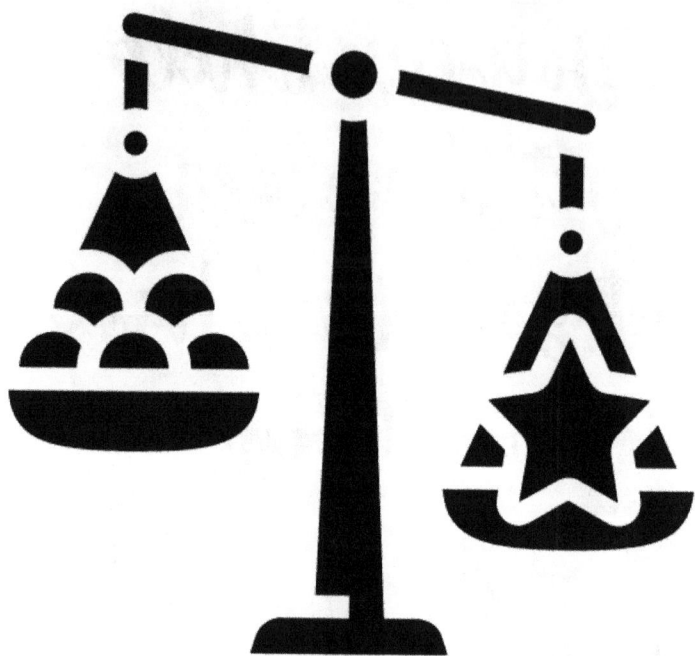

AGING WELL

#1
YOUR MIND DECIDES YOUR FATE WHEN IT COMES TO AGING GRACEFULLY.

WHY NOT EMBRACE IT WITH A HEALTHY OUTLOOK?

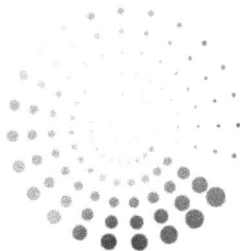

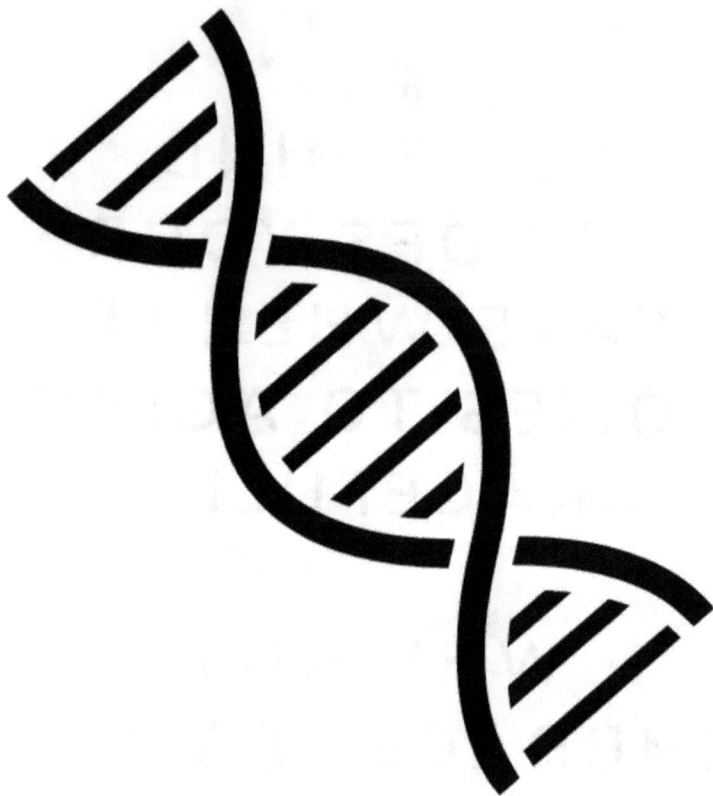

NO GUARANTEES

#2

DIET & LIFESTYLE CHOICES DRIVE OUR CELLULAR FUNCTION OR DYSFUNCTION, NOT GENETICS.

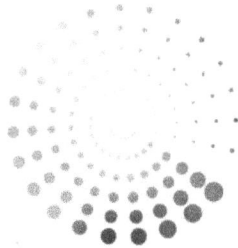

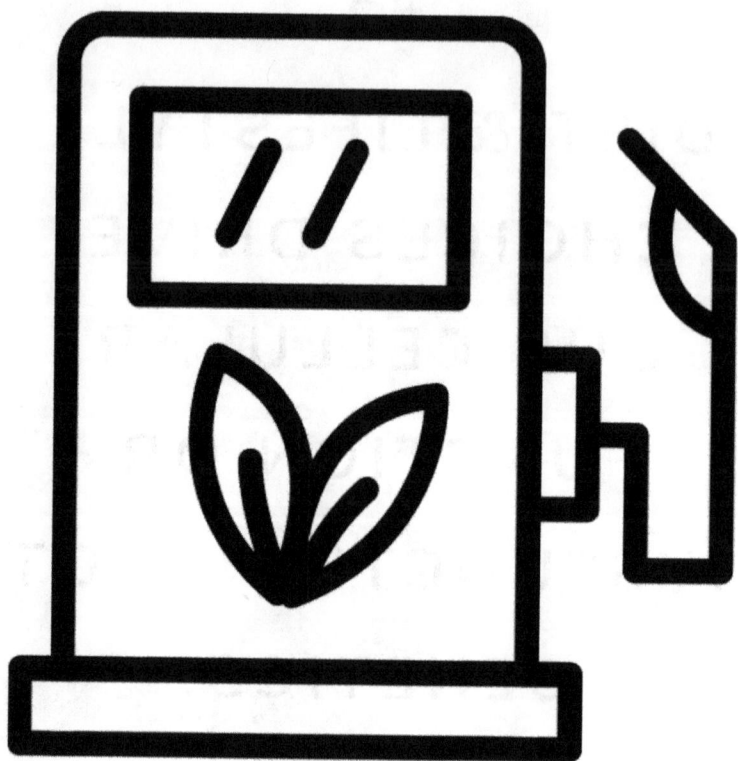

QUALITY FUEL

#3
QUALITY FOODS CREATE QUALITY FUEL FOR OUR CELLS TO FUNCTION PROPERLY.

JUNK IN= JUNK OUT

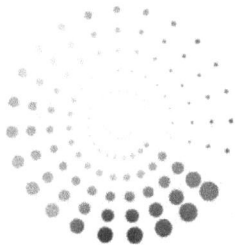

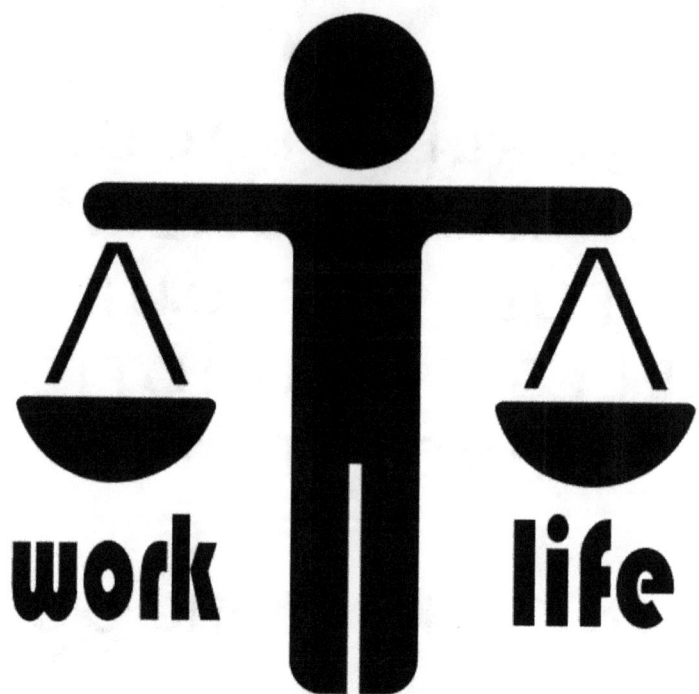

work life

FIND
BALANCE

#4

FOCUS ON LIVING A LIFESTYLE THAT SUPPORTS LESS STRESS, QUALITY SLEEP, EXERCISE AND POSITIVITY.

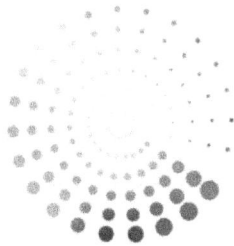

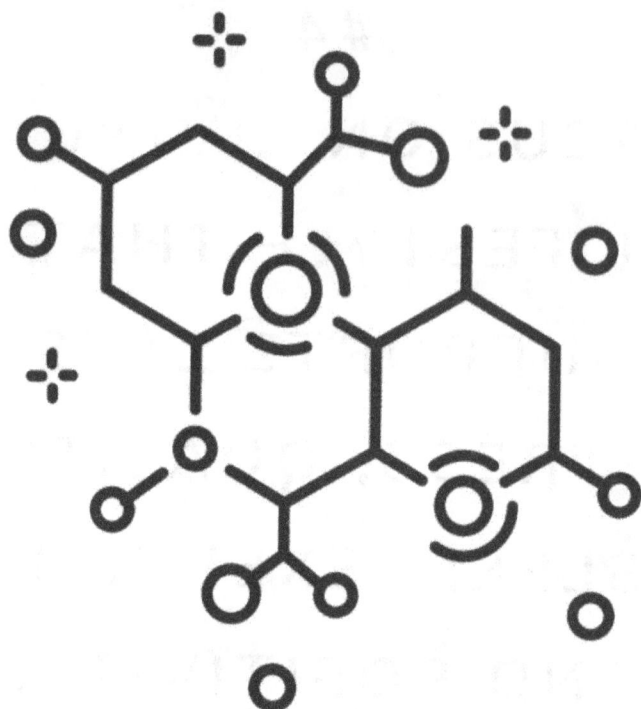

CELLULAR
LONGEVITY

#5

OPTIMIZE YOUR CELLULAR RESILIENCE WITH VARIOUS FORMS OF BIOHACKING.

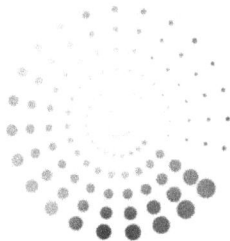

mindset

MASTER EMOTIONS FOR OPTIMAL HEALTH

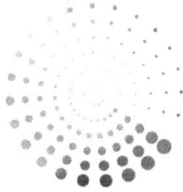

"Your body hears everything your mind says."

—NAOMI JUDD

Our mindset has a profound impact on our life's trajectory, influencing love, success, happiness, and most importantly our health. Many focus on diet and exercise as the primary paths to well-being, and these are of course important. But the real battleground often lies within our minds. Our thoughts are powerful catalysts, triggering reactions at the cellular level that can set in motion positive or negative sequences.

Our thoughts affect our health—a truth I discovered through personal experience. While I'd heard about the mind-body connection for years and even practiced positive mantras, I didn't truly understand their impact. What I didn't realize was that my private thoughts about my health were being absorbed by my body at a cellular level, creating unconscious patterns that shaped my wellbeing.

EMOTIONAL VS. MENTAL HEALTH

It's crucial to understand that emotional health and mental health, while related, are not identical. As licensed psychologist Juli Fraga, PsyD, explains, emotional health "focuses on being in tune with our emotions, vulnerability, and authenticity." Mental health encompasses our emotional, psychological, and social well-being, influencing how we think, feel and behave, and how we handle stress.

Our mindset shapes our physical health through both conscious and unconscious thoughts, influencing our body at the cellular level.

Good emotional health is fundamental to fostering resilience, self-awareness and contentment. It's important to note that good emotional health doesn't mean being happy all the time or being free of negative emotions. We're human, after all. Instead, it's about having the skills and resources to manage life's challenges in a way that promotes a healthier cellular environment.

MINDFULNESS: A KEY TO EMOTIONAL HEALTH

Mindfulness involves three key elements:

1. Being aware
2. Being mindful
3. Paying attention purposefully and without judgment

Practicing mindfulness can be as simple as focusing on one task at a time, taking a break from social media, or turning routine chores into mental breaks. The key is consistency. Dedicating even a few minutes a day to mindfulness can make a significant difference.

CONTROLLING OUR EMOTIONS

Uncontrolled emotions like anxiety and chronic worry can have detrimental effects on our health. A constant state of anxiety not only drains our adrenal glands but also creates negative vibrations at the cellular level. This persistent fight-or-flight state can wreak havoc on our bodies if it becomes chronic.

Consider this example. If you have coronary artery disease (CAD), your heart may be deprived of oxygen. This deprivation, called myocardial ischemia, occurs in 30 to 50% of all CAD patients and can be exacerbated by emotional stress. In fact, for those with any type of heart disease, strong emotions like anger can cause severe and even fatal irregular heart rhythms.

The expressions "died from fright" and "worried to death" aren't just figures of speech—they reflect real physiological possibilities. Furthermore, when patients newly diagnosed with heart disease become depressed, it increases their risk of experiencing a harmful heart-related event within the year.

This information isn't meant to instill fear, but to create *awareness*. Our emotions are powerful modulators of our health, and understanding this connection is crucial for maintaining our overall well-being.

PERSONAL STORY

In 2011, my husband and I visited my neurologist, desperately seeking treatment for my deteriorating muscles. Instead, we received devastating news. The doctor diagnosed me with nonspecific ALS, also known as ALS of unknown etiology. When we asked what could be done, his blunt response was chilling: nothing. Make her comfortable, call EMS for seizures and choking, and start looking into nursing homes or long-term care. (Word to the wise: If you're diagnosed with a condition like ALS and don't have prior insurance for nursing home care, you may not get coverage.)

Throughout my health journey, I rarely cried. I always believed answers were out there, and that God's purpose was what mattered most. But this time was different. The finality of the diagnosis, the absence of hope, weighed on me like never before. As we sat in stunned silence in our car, my tears finally fell. Was this it? Had Western medicine finally beaten me down to this grim existence?

The thought of telling our boys, then aged 12 and 16, seemed inconceivable. I couldn't muster my usual "we got this" attitude but in the same breath I was not about to give in either.

We drove home in silence, another busy afternoon ahead with a basketball game to attend. There was no time for processing. We stuffed our emotions, put on brave faces, and functioned as if nothing had happened. Before we got home, I told my husband, "This is not how it's going to end. Don't listen to the doctor. Let me process this, and I'll figure out our next steps."

This was my lowest point. The weight of the diagnosis felt like an elephant on my shoulders. Even through my bout with throat cancer, I'd never allowed myself to feel the full gravity of bad news for long. My mantra had always been that becoming emotional only prevents you from moving forward. "There's no crying in baseball," right?

But I knew God wouldn't abandon me. As dire as the circumstances were, I reminded myself that doctors are human. They make mistakes and can't control our destiny. When I finally gathered myself, I decided that my neurologist had simply given us his best guess. My job now was to focus on staying alive and keeping my faith. Death would not be my destination.

After allowing myself to grieve and process this unimaginable news, it was time to adjust my mindset. Rather than succumbing to the circumstance, I decided to seek out a doctor who could provide answers. My focus, mindset and determination, coupled with God's mercy and strength, gave me the willpower to persevere. Had I simply accepted the prognosis that was handed to me I would have never looked elsewhere for answers. My boys' lives would have changed forever and I would have indeed ended up dying an ugly and painful death never knowing the root cause was in one of my binders all along. Because of my mindset and strong will to live, I was able to find a doctor and the path to recovery. The mind is a powerful tool few of us know how to use, mine saved my life.

How many people resolve themselves to the first diagnosis they hear? Maybe that's you or your loved one or a friend? Answers are out there if you have a strong mindset and will to live beyond any prognosis given.

"When you go through deep waters, I will be with you. And, when you go through rivers of difficulty, you will not drown. When you walk through the fire of oppression you will not be burned up, the flames will not consume you."

—ISAIAH 43:2

GOOD VIBES = GOOD HEALTH

Our thoughts have powerful health implications that aren't always immediately apparent. The effects can be cumulative, building over time. Repeating negative thoughts, whether subconscious or conscious, can create new neural pathways that perpetuate a cycle of negativity without our awareness.

At a cellular level, our thoughts have vibrational energy. "Good vibes" isn't just slang—it represents a state of being we should all strive for. This positive energy constitutes our personal energy field and fuels us at a cellular level. These vibrations are rhythms within us that facilitate cellular communication.

Our bodies exhibit various physiological rhythms we can easily observe and measure, such as heartbeats, breathing rates, and circadian rhythms. However, there are much smaller vibrations occurring within our bodies as well. Inside each of our cells, molecules vibrate at characteristic rates.

Warning: Scientific information ahead. If this isn't your area of interest, feel free to skip to the bold text.

Before my chronic illness, I was studying to become a registered nurse and to potentially pursue a physician's assistant license. I had research aspirations in the field of molecular immunology.

This background reflects my fascination with the cellular processes involved in alternative therapies.

From a molecular perspective, vibrations play a crucial role in our body's functioning. Using atomic-force microscopes, researchers have detected molecules' nanoscale vibrations—much smaller than one one-thousandth the diameter of a human hair. These vibrations generate electromagnetic energy waves that can cause changes in our cells, affecting how our body functions.

Different molecules vibrate at various rates, and these rates can be influenced by environmental conditions like temperature.

So what's the connection between thoughts, behaviors, and vibrations?

Research has long shown that **thoughts and behaviors affect the rhythms in your body**. For instance, anxious thoughts trigger the release of stress hormones and alter your heart rate variability or HRV. Similarly, musical vibrations can affect thoughts, emotions, and body systems. Musical vibrations affect mood through several mechanisms; fast beats can create excitement or happiness this is known as emotional resonance. Music can also trigger physiological changes altering breathing patterns, which can then influence feelings of anxiety or relaxation. Engaging music can also promote mindfulness helping you to focus on the present moment and reduce stress.

Vibrational energy experts propose that our behaviors and thoughts can alter smaller rhythms even at the cellular and atomic levels. **In essence, changing your thoughts has the potential to change your emotional state and influence your overall health.** While these molecular vibrations are tiny, their effects can be significant.

The field of energy medicine is expanding, offering various modalities to support the body's healing processes. These include red light therapy, infrared therapy, and PEMF technology, all of which affect the body at the cellular level.

While research on the benefits of vibrational energy is still developing, many associated techniques have well-documented health benefits.

Here are a few ways to incorporate healing at the vibrational level:

- Prayer
- Deep breathing
- Meditation
- Acupuncture
- Chakra balancing
- Yoga
- Grounding or earthing
- Consuming plant-based foods
- Practicing gratitude
- PEMF therapy
- Red and infrared light therapy
- Vibrational sound therapy

TRAUMA AND PTSD

Learning to cope with negative experiences that are stored in our subconscious can be critical to overcoming our hurdles with health and healing. When your body is constantly in a state of "readiness" or high alert, you are overusing our sympathetic nervous system. There is never a time when you don't feel "on"— and it's exhausting. For my part, multiple head traumas and traumatic accidents have left me with debilitating post-traumatic stress disorder (PTSD) at times, so I can attest to this exhausting state of being. Let's just say I'm not a great passenger in a car, but I'm working on it!

If not managed, this fight-or-flight state triggers a downward health spiral with numerous symptoms and conditions: suppression of our immune system, blood sugar dysfunction, decreased libido, hormonal imbalance and infertility. It can also slow digestion and affect the gut microbiome, which then leads to poor sleep, constant fatigue and so on.

Regulating our nervous system so we can break free from this constant state of alertness begins with mindfulness. This might include meditation, as we've discussed, psychotherapy, hypnosis, or programs like HeartMath®, which focus on heart rate variability training, the ability to slow down or speed up our heart beats per minute along with coherence practices to enhance emotional resilience and reduce stress.

Something I've learned about recently is perception reframing, a cognitive technique used to change the way one interprets a situation, event or experience. A software called Evox measures voice inflection and gathers information through a galvanic hand sensor while a person speaks about a topic they wish to change their perceptions about. This voice energy is then plotted into a perception index, which gives the client a visual image of their perception. The person then meditates on the topic until their perception shifts at both a conscious and subconscious level. By altering the way you perceive something, you can effectively shift your emotional responses and behaviors.

There are other methods of adjusting your mindset and emotional responses—this chapter is not an exhaustive list! But it indicates the possibilities, and of the power of the mind when we guide it in a direction that supports true health.

YUSUF'S STORY

During my second visit to True North Health Center's fasting clinic, I met Yusuf S. Saleem on day 27 of his 30-day water fast. A tall, thin Muslim man who had lost almost 30 pounds, Yusuf possessed an enthusiastic sense of humor and—at 72 years of age —a lifetime of knowledge that I thoroughly enjoyed. His presence of mind and powerful mindset drew me into every conversation we had.

Yusuf's health journey began with a stage-one prostate cancer diagnosis. Faced with the standard treatment options of radiation, drugs, and possible surgery, he chose a different path. Driven by his faith, positive mindset, and determination, Yusuf decided to try water fasting to heal his body naturally.

Having previously attempted a 13-day water-only fast at home, Yusuf was familiar with fasting's healing potential. His ability to fast for so long independently is admirable—and something I wouldn't attempt without medical supervision.

Yusuf had traveled from Philadelphia to Santa Rosa, California, bringing with him an unwavering positive attitude. His triumph through the fasting process was inspiring. Even on day 29, he was still laughing and joking, a self-proclaimed "chatterbox" with seemingly endless knowledge.

Yusuf expressed profound gratitude daily for the opportunity and ability to address his cancer with water fasting (please always consult your doctor prior to engaging in any treatment, such as fasting. This is a medically supervised program, and each patient is fully vetted prior to entering the program, this is not a recommendation or suggestion for cancer treatment.).

Despite Yusuf's numerous challenges, advanced age, cancer diagnosis and obvious food deprivation he was always full of light and hope, he focused on his future rather than dwelling on the moment, potential treatments or prognosis. His mindset, coupled with constant prayer and gratitude, maximized the benefits of his thirty day fast.

His bright spirit touched many lives at True North. Yusuf looks forward to continuing his work as a methadone counselor, and he feels blessed by this opportunity for reflection and renewal. The world is undoubtedly a better place with his presence, and I feel fortunate to have shared this experience with him.

MEDITATION

Meditation, an ancient practice dating back thousands of years, has gained worldwide recognition for its benefits to brain health and well-being. As modern technology advances, researchers continue to uncover how and why meditation is so effective.

There are numerous forms of meditation, both religious and secular, including yoga and transcendental meditation. Despite their differences, all share a common goal: to quiet the mind and focus energy.

"Evidence is the loudest voice"

—DR. JOE DISPENZA, MEDITATION EXPERT

In groundbreaking studies, scientists have explored what happens when we close our eyes, go within, and connect to our energy source. Using protocols similar to pharmaceutical studies, researchers from the University of California San Diego extracted data from thousands of participants at Dr. Joe Dispenza's retreats worldwide—with profound results.

We are not bound by our genes or self-limiting behaviors. Our subconscious controls 85% of our daily behavior and predicts our reactions to external stimuli. By age six, 95% of our automatic subconscious thoughts have been programmed, forming the root of our behavior mechanisms for life.

The good news is these pre-programmed behaviors can be altered through meditation, which can improve our stress response and offers many health benefits. Meditation modulates our stress response by creating new tissue and blood environments that enhance health and resilience.

During guided meditation, research has shown that cell behavior of neurons can be manipulated during high-energy surges. According to Dr. Dispenza, our cells comprise 99% energy and just 1% matter.

Can we create and affect biological processes in our bodies through thought alone? The possibility of manipulating cell behavior through meditation is a powerful tool worth exploring. The potential is exciting!

Thyroid Story

Dr. Joe Dispenza, the author of *Evolve Your Brain: The Science of Changing Your Mind* shared a story about the healing power of the mind that I'd like to share with you. A high-achieving businesswoman collapsed one day due to chest tightness. At the ER, she was told she needed to remove her thyroid or risk a heart attack. Despite her reservations, she eventually had the surgery.

Afterward, she began daily meditations, visualizing her thyroid growing back healthier than before. She followed Dr. Dispenza's program and believed in its effectiveness. When she returned for a checkup, her doctor was puzzled by her lab results and referred her back to the surgeon.

The surgeon, skeptical of the lab results, performed an ultrasound on the area where her thyroid had been removed. To his shock, he discovered her thyroid had regrown. He confirmed this by comparing the ultrasound to post-surgery X-rays that showed the thyroid's absence.

This surprising story opens our minds to the possibilities of the power of meditation and visualization and You don't have anything to lose—and potentially you have a lot to gain—by adding meditation and mindfulness to your vitality toolset.

ACTIONS YOU CAN TAKE TODAY

Implement these five strategies into your daily routine:

1. **EMOTION CONTROL**: Emotions drive everything happening in the body. Practicing mindfulness and awareness are keys to resilience.

2. **HEALTHY RESPONSE**: Learn coping mechanisms that help you Respond instead of React to situations.
3. **MOVE IT OR LOSE IT**: Fifteen minutes of movement releases "feel good" hormones knowns as endorphins.
4. **GOOD VIBES**: Incorporate positive thoughts and energy daily to build healthier cells.
5. **DEEP SLEEP**: Quality sleep equals being less vulnerable to stress, anxiety or runaway emotions. Deep sleep also allows our immune system to go into repair mode.

"It is not the trials in your life that develop or destroy you, but rather your response to those hardships."

—DR. CHARLES STANLEY

"your body hears everything your mind says."

-Naomi Judd

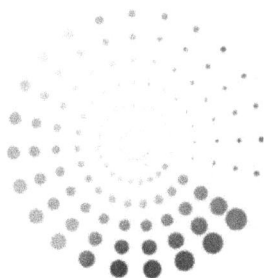

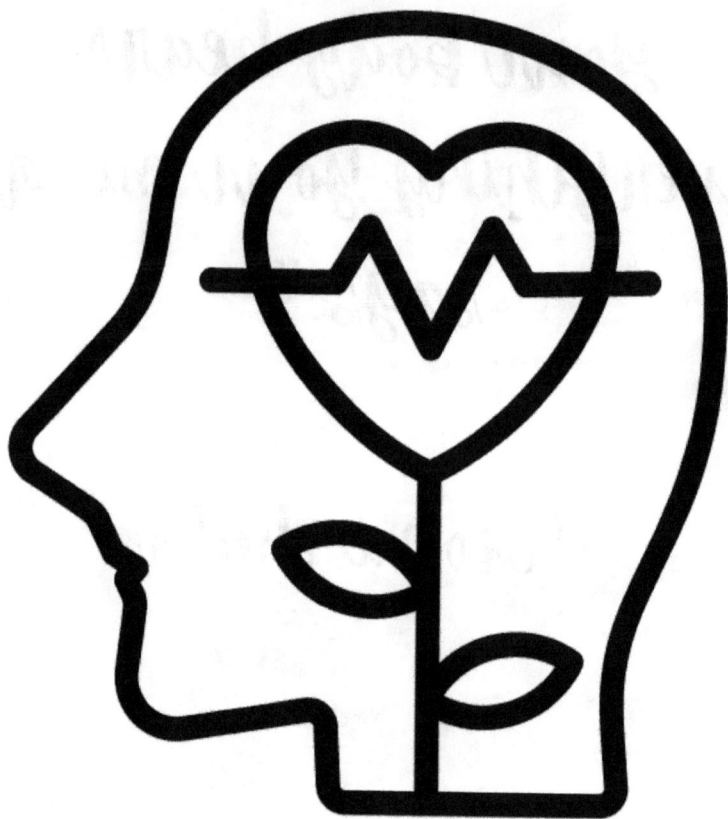

EMOTION
CONTROL

#1
EMOTIONS DRIVE EVERYTHING HAPPENING IN THE BODY.

PRACTICING MINDFULNESS & AWARENESS ARE KEYS TO RESILIENCE.

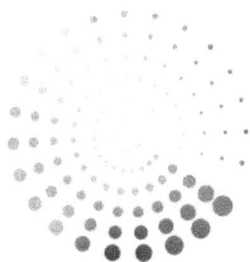

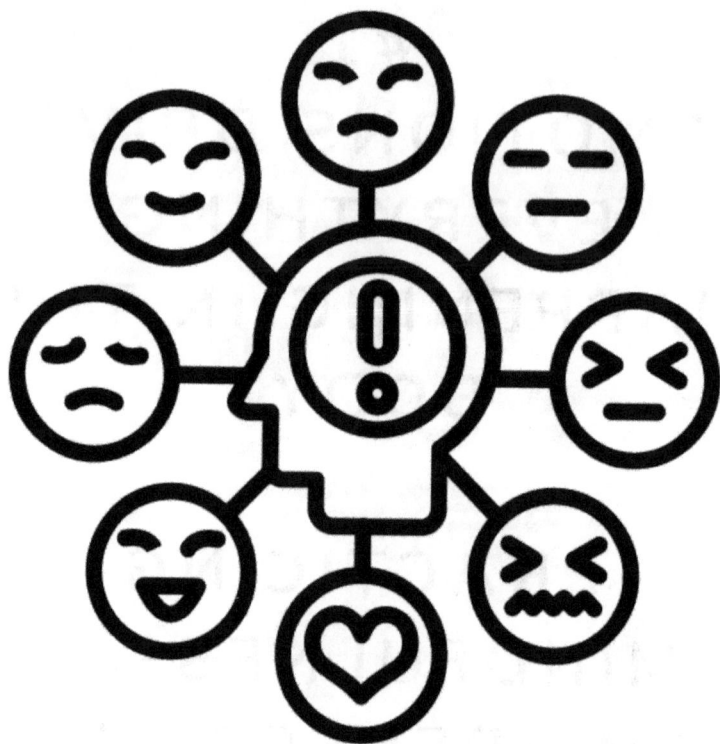

HEALTHY
RESPONSE

#2

LEARN COPING MECHANISMS THAT HELP YOU *RESPOND* INSTEAD OF *REACT* TO SITUATIONS.

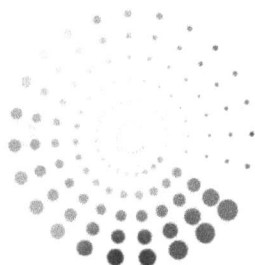

15

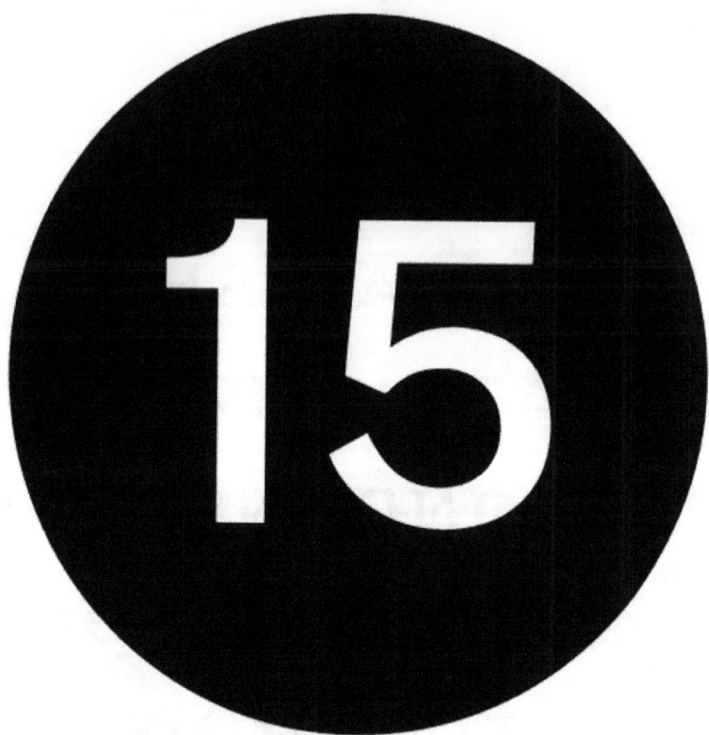

MOVE IT
OR LOSE IT

#3

FIFTEEN MINUTES OF MOVEMENT RELEASES "FEEL GOOD" HORMONES, AKA ENDORPHINES.

WANT TO CHANGE YOUR MOOD, MOVE YOUR BODY!

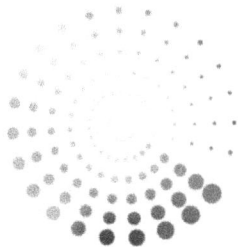

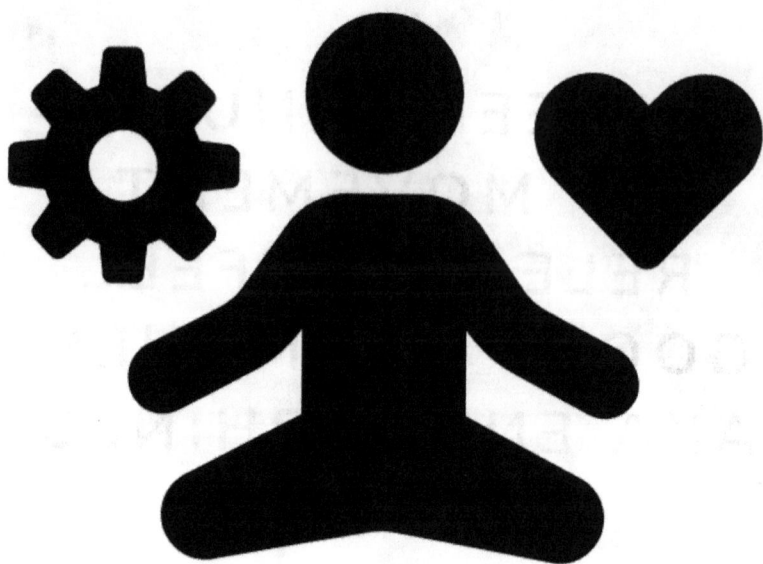

GOOD VIBES

#4
INCORPORATE POSITIVE THOUGHTS & ENERGY DAILY TO BUILD HEALTHIER CELLS.

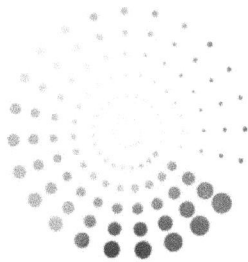

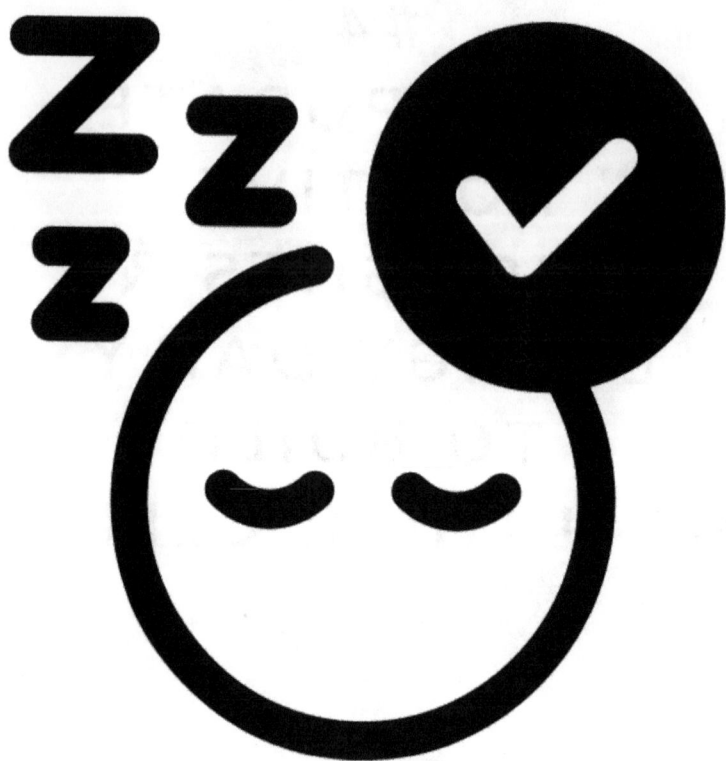

DEEP SLEEP

#5
QUALITY SLEEP=
BEING LESS
VULNERABLE TO
STRESS, ANXIETY
OR RUNAWAY
EMOTIONS.

DEEP SLEEP ALSO
ALLOWS OUR
IMMUNE SYSTEM TO
GO INTO REPAIR
MODE.

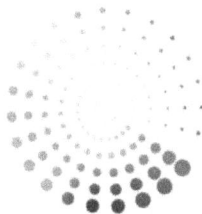

conclusion

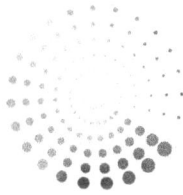

As the old saying goes, "The only thing guaranteed in life is death." Morbid, but true. So how we get from life to death is up to us. The upside, as I like to say, is that it is possible to live our lives, our *entire lives*, with *vitality*!

My challenge to you is to ask yourself... What is *your* priority? Where do *your* health and vitality fall on the scale of what's important? Do you prefer to pay endless medical bills, waste precious hours at the doctor's office, or spend money on drugs that complicate matters but never get to the root of the problem?

Our lives can be complicated: full of stress, toxins and bad influences, from processed food to the barrage of pharmaceutical ads that claim to cure one thing but then turn around and give you five more conditions. Where do *you* want to draw the line? Simply being *reactive* to our circumstances can be exhausting, and it gets us nowhere.

In my experience, it is far easier, less time-consuming and way cheaper to be *proactive* about your health. You've taken the first step by picking up this book and being curious about other possibilities. I hope that you've learned enough to *act on your own behalf*—before you are debilitated by disease or chronic illness. *Your health is your greatest asset.*

Time is a precious gift you can't get back once you've wasted it. *You* are worth the time and effort it takes to live an optimally healthy life now. Why wait?

Change is not easy, and perfection is not the expectation here. You've built a lifestyle that you are comfortable with and used to. That lifestyle is like a house of bricks, every choice is a brick on that foundation. Changing your lifestyle or habits will involve removing one brick at time to incorporate a stronger, healthier foundation.

A word of advice from someone who did not always treat herself with compassion: be kind to yourself through the process. It isn't easy, but it is doable! Focus on your end goal—your health—set goals, and choose to conquer one thing at a time from the "Action Steps" section that follows. This is *your* journey and no one else's.

I pray these health tools and stories have inspired you to take charge of your health today. If this book opened your eyes to even one alternative, I'm grateful. I hope the information provided blessed you in some way and that it will have a ripple effect so that communities become more open to the possibilities that are out there.

I love connecting with people, so if you have any questions or just want to share your story, I would love to hear from you!

Would you help someone struggling with health issues if it was easy, free, and took only a minute? Here are three simple ways you can make a meaningful difference in someone's life:

1. Share your experience: Leave a quick book review online to help others find this book
2. Pass it on: Lend your copy to someone who might need this inspiration
3. Share the knowledge: Tell someone you care about one health tip you learned reading this book.

Remember: Ideas are one of the few things you can give away—and still keep!

Do you want to join my mission and transform lives through wellness? Email me to learn how I can help you open a successful health spa in your area.

Ready to continue your wellness journey? Visit www.thevitalityso lutionbook.com to access our vibrant community, discover the latest research, and learn about upcoming Vitality Retreats and events.

With deep appreciation and gratitude,

Carey Mencarini
Founder, IV Lounge and Liv Optimal

CONNECT WITH ME!

Email: Carey@livoptimalnow.com
IV Lounge—IV Drip Bar and Health spa

Join our wellness mission!

Open a health spa in your area—email me to learn more. www.ivlounge-edh.com

Liv Optimal—Health and Wellness Company www. livoptimalnow.com

The Vitality Solution Program and Retreats: www.thevitalitysolu-tionbook.com

action steps

Ready to put these Action Steps into practice? I've transformed them into beautifully designed Vitality Action Cards to keep you inspired and on track!

Download your free PDF and display these eye-catching reminders wherever you need motivation—by your desk, on your bathroom mirror, or in your wellness journal. These cards make the vital practices we've explored simple to remember and implement daily.

Want to share your wellness journey? Send me a photo of your cards in their new home! Grab your free Vitality Action Cards now (for a limited time): www.thevitalitysolutionbook.com/gifts

THE
VITALITY
Solution

Recharge your health with IV Vitamin Therapy, Mindfulness, Fasting, and more!

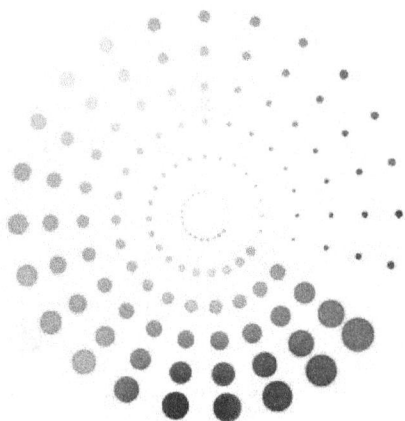

CAREY MENCARINI
Foreword by Aurora Winter, MBA

ACTION STEP
CARD DECK

THE VITALITY SOLUTION: ACTION STEPS

IMMUNITY

1. **WHO'S DRIVING**: Remember you are in control, not your genes.
2. **FOR YOUR MIND & IMMUNITY**: Increase fiber-rich foods & decrease the inflammatory ones.
3. **LIFESTYLE OPTIMIZATION**: Get quality sleep, limit daily stress and reduce toxin exposure.
4. **KNOW YOUR SUPERPOWER**: Be aware of the signals before your body gets depleted.
5. **MAINTAIN NUTRIENT BALANCE**: Supplement high-quality vitamins daily, as needed.

DETOX

1. **KNOW YOUR ENVIRONMENT**: Be aware of what you ingest, inhale and absorb, knowledge is power.
2. **PAY ATTENTION TO THE SIGNS**: Listen to your body, pay attention to symptoms of toxin overload.
3. **ENVIRONMENTAL DETOX**: Filter your air/water, eat clean foods and lessen EMF exposure.
4. **INTERNAL DETOX**: Incorporate physical methods of detoxification through various methods or supplements.

RESTORE

1. **DISEASE OR DEFICIENCY**: Do your homework, sometimes symptoms can be our body's cry for vitamins.

2. **QUALITY NOT QUANTITY**: Choose high-quality vitamins based on your needs, not your neighbors.

3. **OPTIMAL LEVELS, OPTIMAL LIFE**: Maintain adequate levels of nutrients every day. As the demands of life increase so does the bodies need for nutrition.

4. **CONSISTENCY IS KEY**: Regular supplementation is essential for optimal health. Toxins, daily stress and life can deplete us of vital nutrients.

LONGEVITY

1. **AGING WELL**: Your mind decides your fate when it comes to aging gracefully. Why not embrace it with a healthy outlook?

2. **NO GUARANTEES**: Diet and lifestyle choice drive our cellular function or dysfunction, not our genes.

3. **QUALITY FUEL**: Quality foods create quality fuel for our cells to function properly. Junk in = Junk out!

4. **FIND BALANCE**: Focus on living a lifestyle that supports less stress, quality sleep, exercise and positivity.

5. **CELLULAR LONGEVITY**: Optimize your cellular resilience with various forms of biohacking.

MINDSET

1. **EMOTION CONTROL**: Emotions drive everything happening in the body. Practicing mindfulness and awareness are keys to resilience.

2. **HEALTHY RESPONSE**: Learn coping mechanisms that help you Respond instead of React to situations.

3. **MOVE IT OR LOSE IT**: Fifteen minutes of movement releases "Feel Good" hormones known as endorphins.

4. **GOOD VIBES**: Incorporate positive thoughts and energy daily to build healthier cells.

5. **DEEP SLEEP**: Quality sleep = being less vulnerable to stress, anxiety or runaway emotions. Deep sleep also allows our immune system to go into repair mode.

resources

Want to stay connected with the latest advances in health and vitality? I'm constantly exploring and validating new therapies, tools, and research to support your wellness journey. Visit www.thevitalitysolutionbook.com/resources for:

- Innovative research and discoveries
- Trusted product recommendations
- Transformative books and documentaries
- Upcoming Vitality Solution events
- Special offers and promotions

Everything I share has been tested and proven effective. I do the research so you can focus on what matters—your health!

RESOURCES BY CHAPTER

CHAPTER 3: IMMUNITY

Genetics vs. Lifestyle—research from Dr. Mark Davis: https://med. stanford.edu/davislab/Research.html

CHAPTER 4: DETOXIFICATION

The Standard American Diet (SAD): https://nutritionfacts.org/ topics/standard-american-diet/

Sandy Cohen, "If You Want to Boost Immunity, Look to the Gut" *UCLA Health* (2021): https://www.uclahealth.org/news/article/ want-to-boost-immunity-look-to-the-gut

Dr. Joseph Pizzorno, *The Toxin Solution: How Hidden Poisons in the Air, Water, Food and Products We Use Are Destroying Our Health—And What We Can Do to Fix It* (2017)

Rebel Health (website): https://rebelhealth.co/

James Colquhoun and Laurentine ten Bosch, *Food Matters* (documentary, 2008): https://www.foodmatters.com/films

World Health Organization (WHO), "Radiation: Electromagnetic Fields" (2026): https://www.who.int/news-room/questions-and-answers/item/radiation-electromagnetic-fields

Credible alternative information about Lyme Disease: https:// www.lymedisease.org/

International Lyme and Associated Diseases Society: https:// www.ilads.org/

CHAPTER 5: RESTORE

Ali Niklewich *et al.*, "The Importance of Vitamin B_{12} for Individuals Choosing Plant-Based Diets," *European Journal of Nutrition* 62 (2023): https://pmc.ncbi.nlm.nih.gov/articles/PMC10030528/

US Institute of Medicine dietary reference intakes for vitamins and minerals: https://pubmed.ncbi.nlm.nih.gov/23193625/

Cleveland Clinic, "Signs You May Have a Magnesium Deficiency" (2022): https://health.clevelandclinic.org/feeling-fatigued-could-it-be-magnesium-deficiency-and-if-so-what-to-do-about-it

National Institutes of Health (NIH), governmental guidelines for Recommended Daily Intake (RDI): https://ods.od.nih.gov/Health-Information/nutrientrecommendations.aspx

CHAPTER 6: LONGEVITY

Dr. Joe Dispenza: https://drjoedispenza.com/scientific-research

Food transit times: https://www.wellandgood.com/

Dr. Mindy Pelz, *Fast Like a Girl: A Woman's Guide to Using the Healing Power of Fasting to Burn Fat, Boost Energy, and Balance Hormones* (2022): https://drmindypelz.com/

Blue Zones: https://www.bluezones.com/

World Health Organization (WHO), "Air Pollution": https://www.who.int/health-topics/air-pollution

National Institute on Aging: https://www.nia.nih.gov/

Nicotinamide Adenine Dinucleotide (NAD) studies

Dina Radenkovic *et al.*, "Clinical Evidence for Targeting NAD Therapeutically" *Pharmaceuticals* (2020): https://pmc.ncbi.nlm.nih.gov/articles/PMC7558103/

Naidy Brady and Yue Liu, "NAD+ Therapy in Age-Related Degenerative Disorders," *Experimental Gerontology* (2020): https://pubmed.ncbi.nlm.nih.gov/31917996/

Dylan G. Arrazati, "NAD+ Is 'The Future' of Longevity: What Celebrities Are Doing to 'Never Age'," *NAD+ Aging Science* (2024): https://www.nad.com/news/nad-is-the-future-of-longevity-what-celebrities-are-doing-to-never-age

Sarah Handzel "Is NAD therapy all it's cracked up to be? Here's the evidence" MDLinx (2022): https://www.mdlinx.com/article/is-nad-therapy-all-its-cracked-up-to-be-heres-the-evidence/4nto35HwTjVcM6Y9J3anaF

Lloyd Burrell, *Electric Sense*: https://www.electricsense.com/

CHAPTER 7: MINDSET

Mayo Clinic, "Positive Thinking: Stop Negative Self-Talk to Reduce Stress" (2023): https://www.mayoclinic.org/healthy-lifestyle/stress-management/in-depth/positive-thinking/art-20043950

"What is Mindfulness?" *Mindful* (2020): https://www.mindful.org/what-is-mindfulness/

Julie Corliss, "Mindfulness Meditation May Ease Anxiety, Mental Stress," *Harvard Health Blog* (2014): https://www.health.harvard.edu/blog/mindfulness-meditation-may-ease-anxiety-mental-stress-201401086967

Nick Earl, "The Science Behind Frequency Healing: How Can Frequencies Impact Health?" *HealthVibed* (2024): https://healthvibed.com/the-science-behind-frequency-healing-how-can-frequencies-impact-health/

"Dr. Joe Dispenza on Neuroscience and the Quantum Field," *Worgia Writes* (2024): https://worgia.substack.com/p/dr-joe-dispenza-on-neuroscience-and

National Center for Complementary and Integrative Health, "Meditation and Mindfulness: Effectiveness and Safety" (2022): https://nccih.nih.gov/health/meditation/overview.htm

Matthew Thorpe and Rachael Ajmera, "How Meditation Benefits Your Mind and Body," *Healthline* (2024): https://www.healthline.com/nutrition/12-benefits-of-meditation

Dr. Joe Dispenza, Author, Researcher and Meditation Expert.: https://drjoedispenza.com/

Ready to take your journey to vibrant health even further?

I've created exclusive bonus gifts to support your success! Get instant access at: www.thevitalitysolutionbook.com/gifts

Plus, join our wellness community to receive:

- Early access to my upcoming companion workbook
- In-depth guides on specialized health topics
- Latest research and *break*through discoveries
- Exclusive content and special offers

Let's make this your year of extraordinary health and vitality. Start your transformation today!

www.thevitalitysolutionbook.com

acknowledgments

First and foremost, I want to acknowledge my Lord and Savior Jesus Christ. Without my Christian faith and miraculous divine interventions on more than one occasion, I would not be here to write this today. My daily conversations and walks with God kept me sane and focused as they do still today. There is no substitute for His presence.

I appreciate my earthly father, Johnny Tallant, whose life ended far too soon at the hands of our misguided medical system during COVID. You are loved and missed beyond words.

To my mom, sisters and their families, the Gotelli family, and father-in-law..... for all of your support, love and prayers, I am grateful!

To my amazing village of BFFs Karyn, Kelly, Karen, Rene, Cindy, Robin and Gretchen, who became my mom army during my illness. I have immense appreciation for the hours you spent driving me to IV therapy, ER visits and doctor appointments; for the meals and groceries delivered (before Amazon came along); and for the time you spent babysitting me or the kids so Mike could work.

Your loving friendship and support helped me be a "regular" mom for as long as possible so my boys could have a somewhat normal life during such an unstable time. Your friendship and willingness to walk with me through this lengthy journey truly blessed me and my family in ways you will never know. I am forever grateful!

Dr. Annemieke Austin, your determination to find the root cause of my illnesses saved my life—literally. After others had given up on me, you dredged through my endless binders of records to find the needle in the haystack. I will forever be in your debt. Thank you!

I am immensely grateful for the Sanoviv Medical Institute and Dr. Francisco, my doctor through it all. They were with me from the beginning clear to the end! From its amazing staff to its healing location in Rosarito, Mexico, the clinic is truly a magical place when one is in a health crisis.

For your help, support, and kindness during my health journey, I am so grateful to Dr. Mora, Dr. Hamilton, my friends in the IV department and the awesome staff at Health Associates in Sacramento.

Writing *The Vitality Solution* while running a business and caring for my family seemed daunting until I found Aurora Winter, MBA, founder of www.SamePagePublishing.com. Her kindness, deep listening, skilled coaching, and compassionate guidance made this book possible. I was inspired by her personal story, which in turn gave me the courage to share mine. Through her Spoken Author™ method, she helped transform my health journey into a message of hope. As we refined my message through our interviews and discussions, I watched it become more compelling and powerful. The result is this book, which I believe will help others reclaim their health and vitality.

Lastly, I am grateful to Ha Dang, ND L.Ac, dear friend and business partner, for her belief that I could do the impossible: bring an IV bar to life to help others! Her passion for helping others and her expertise in the field of IV nutrition (among others) continue to inspire me to forge the way despite the constant challenges that face our industry.

about the author

CAREY MENCARINI: ADVOCATE FOR HEALTH, HOPE, AND HEALING

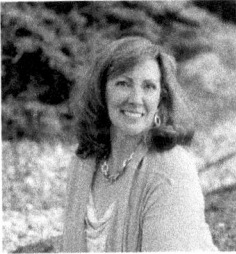

Carey Mencarini

Carey Mencarini, founder of IV Lounge, Liv Optimal, and the Vitality Solution Program & Retreats, transformed her life after battling a devastating diagnosis of Lyme Disease and ALS. Once confined to a wheelchair and given a grim prognosis, Carey refused to accept defeat.

Through unwavering determination and a commitment to alternative medicine, she reclaimed her health and reignited her passion for life. Today, Carey empowers others to embrace natural healing methods, take charge of their well-being, and rediscover their vitality. Her inspiring journey is a testament to the power of resilience and the body's ability to heal when supported with the right tools and mindset.

Get your gifts here: www.thevitalitysolutionbook.com/gifts

www.ivlounge-edh.com

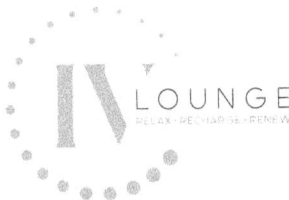

THE
VITALITY
Solution
WORKBOOK

How to Recharge Your Health with
IV Vitamin Therapy, Mindset, Fasting, and More

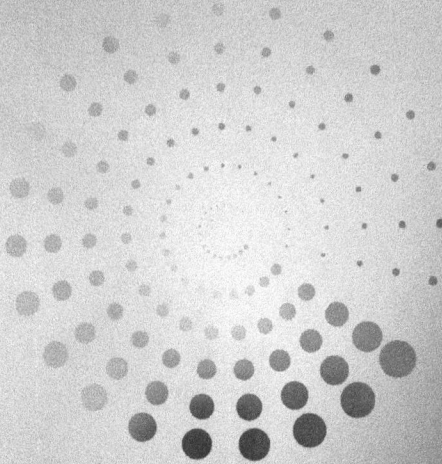

CAREY MENCARINI
Foreword by Aurora Winter, MBA

THE
VITALITY
Solution
IMMUNE SYSTEM

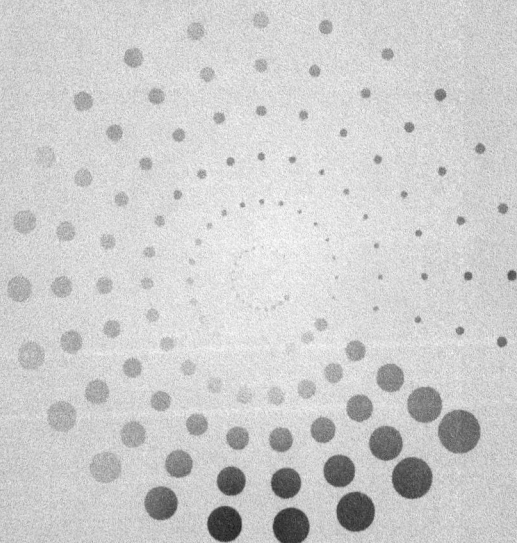

CAREY MENCARINI
Foreword by Aurora Winter, MBA

THE
VITALITY
Solution
DETOX MORE

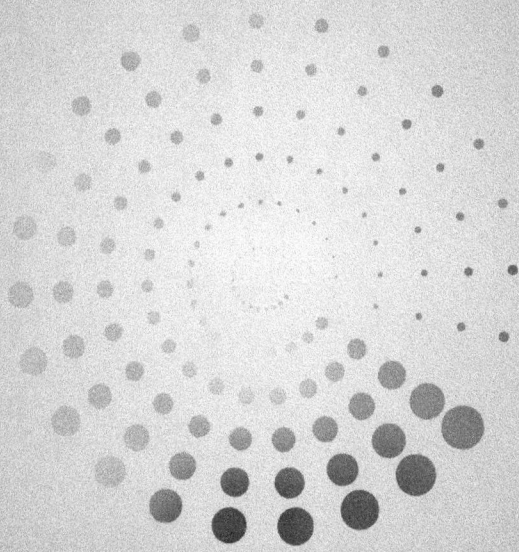

CAREY MENCARINI
Foreword by Aurora Winter, MBA

THE
VITALITY
Solution
RESTORE MORE

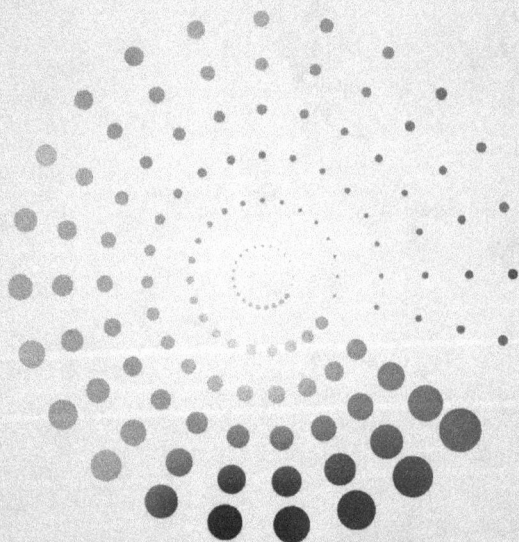

CAREY MENCARINI
Foreword by Aurora Winter, MBA

THE
VITALITY
Solution
LONGEVITY

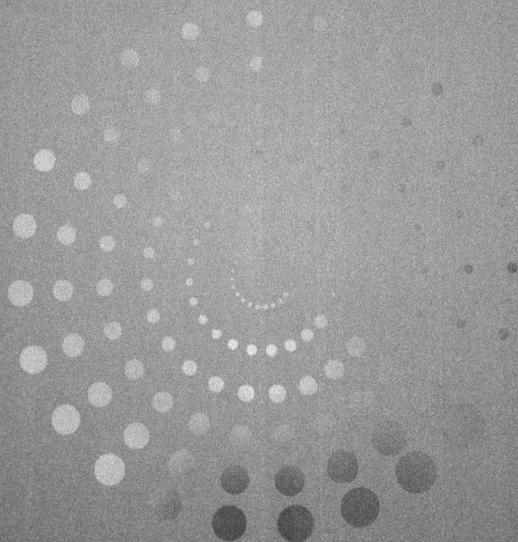

CAREY MENCARINI

Foreword by Aurora Winter, MBA

THE
VITALITY
Solution
MINDSET

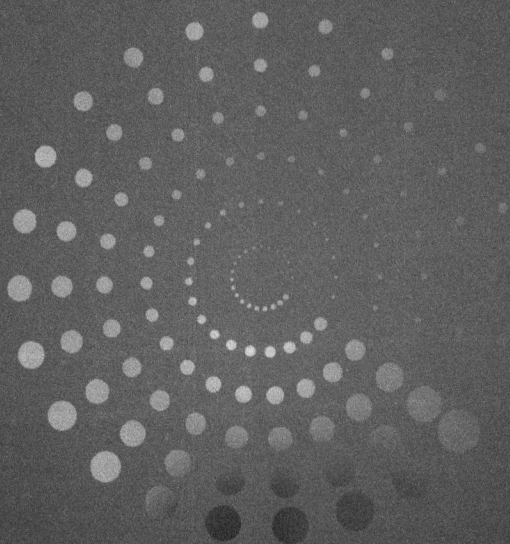

CAREY MENCARINI
Foreword by Aurora Winter, MBA